SAFE &
SOUND

SAFE & SOUND

HOW TO PREVENT AND TREAT THE MOST COMMON CHILDHOOD EMERGENCIES

ELENA BOSQUE, R.N., M.S.

SHEILA WATSON, R.N.

ILLUSTRATIONS BY DIANA THEWLIS

ST. MARTIN'S PRESS
NEW YORK

Note: In the interest of simplicity, the authors have chosen to use masculine pronouns when referring to children and adults of either sex.

DESIGNED BY: SNAP-HAUS GRAPHICS/DIANE STEVENSON

Library of Congress Cataloging in Publication Data

Bosque, Elena.
  Safe and sound : how to prevent and treat the most comon childhood emergencies / Elena Bosque and Sheila Watson.
    p. cm.
  ISBN 0-312-02276-X
  1. Pediatric emergencies.   2. Pediatric emergencies—Prevention.
I. Watson, Sheila, 1950- . II. Title.
RJ370.B67 1988
618.92′0025—dc19

ISBN 0-312-02276-X

10 9 8 7 6 5 4 3 2

This book is dedicated to those people who have reared children successfully, without the support and information that is available today.

Important Note to the Reader

This book should not be used as a substitute for professional medical care or treatment. It is essential that in any medical emergency professional medical care be obtained without unnecessary delay. This book is intended as an introduction to emergency treatment and to promote awareness of various lifesaving techniques; however, a single book such as this cannot provide full or adequate instruction. This book is not a substitute for certification in cardiopulmonary resuscitation (CPR) or other lifesaving methods. It is strongly recommended by the authors, the publisher, and by those at the American Heart Association that every person seek actual training from properly qualified instructors in CPR and other lifesaving techniques. Courses are available in most communities. Call your local hospital, the American Heart Association, or the American Red Cross for information about classes.

CONTENTS

CONTENTS

x

FOREWORD

As the World Health Organization's vision of "health for all by the year 2000" becomes attainable for many countries in the world, it is sobering to remember that only 250 years ago in the so-called developed world, over 60 percent of children never saw their second birthday. With the advent of the Industrial Revolution in Europe and the United States, safety in the home, in the streets, and in the workplace (where many children spent their waking hours) deteriorated. The struggle for survival for many families was so great that child safety had a very low priority, if any at all. It was not until the late nineteenth century that church leaders, writers, sociologists, and public health officers vociferously criticized this callous indifference of business and civic leaders, and the earliest legislation for child protection was passed. With improved housing, sanitation, and water supply, diarrhea and infectious diseases rapidly declined as major causes of infant and childhood mortality; with the advent of immunization and antibiotics, they almost disappeared. Injuries and accidents, however, have *not* decreased as dramatically as infectious diseases, and as Elena Bosque and Sheila Watson point out, they remain high on the list of causes of childhood mortality.

The very word *accident* suggests an element of chance, which implies that an event is neither predictable nor preventable. This is not always true, however, as the excellent section on "Prevention and Treatment of Common Problems" in *Safe & Sound* clearly illustrates.

Until the 1960s the immediate management of a seriously injured child was considered best left to medical professionals, although they are rarely present during an emergency. It was not until closed-chest cardiac massage was shown to be just as effective and much safer than open-chest massage, and until intubation and/or mouth-to-mouth resuscitation replaced emergency tracheotomy, that cardiopulmonary resuscitation (CPR) became the domain of the paramedic, the layperson, and even the parent.

Safe & Sound helps bring the management of serious childhood emergencies into the hands of parents, day-care workers, and other such caregivers. It describes and illustrates the underlying pathophysiologic processes; it simply and clearly outlines the ABCs of emergency care for the child who is choking or

FOREWORD

who has stopped breathing or whose heart has stopped; and it describes in careful detail the immediate care of the poisoned, burned, injured, or drowning child. In addition, the book provides a complete reference section and list of resource materials.

As the authors point out, *Safe & Sound* is in no way meant to replace adequate medical care and advice but rather to provide guidelines during an emergency until professional help can be obtained. Moreover, the authors emphasize that emergency-care skills cannot be learned from a book and that CPR classes (provided by the Red Cross, local fire departments, and the American Heart Association) are essential for all those who care for children.

This small book is a "Dr. Spock" of emergency care for children and, as such, is invaluable for all those who are responsible for children—whether in day-care centers, nursery schools, playgrounds, swimming pools, or at home. Teachers, baby-sitters, grandparents, and most of all parents will want to read and re-read it, for "empowering parents to protect their children's lives . . . helps to increase their sense of control over their own life and destiny" (UNICEF 1988).

June P. Brady, M.D.
University of Nairobi
Kenya

SAFE &
SOUND

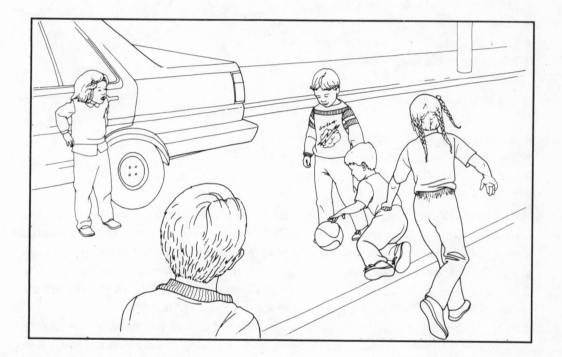

Helping a child grow into a happy, creative, self-reliant individual is one of life's most challenging and rewarding responsibilities. Play is an important factor in a child's growth, but as anyone who takes care of children knows, playtime is also the time when accidents often occur.

Sixty years ago, injuries resulting from accidents caused one out of every ten deaths among infants and children. Today one out of every three childhood deaths is accidental. Accidents are more significant today, because the use of advanced medical technology has decreased the number of deaths caused by common childhood diseases. Even so, the frequency rates are sobering. Each year, almost 10,000 children die from injury due to accidents. Of these:

- 4,000 children die in automobile accidents
- 3,000 children die from poisoning
- 1,600 children die from drowning
- 700 children die from choking.

In addition, each year:

- 250,000 children sustain serious injury from head trauma
- 900 children sustain serious injury from burns
- 40,000 to 50,000 children are permanently disabled by accidental injuries.

We believe that *prevention* is the best defense against childhood accidents. You can learn to protect children from a potentially harmful environment without hindering their growth or their need to explore and play. We hope that you will never need to use any of the emergency lifesaving skills described in the following pages. But knowing these skills and knowing how to respond quickly and effectively in an emergency are essential for your child's welfare, as well as for your peace of mind.

In *Safe & Sound,* you will read about techniques to help you prevent and manage the most common life-threatening emergencies that can occur during infancy and childhood. The instructions follow the guidelines developed by experts at the American Heart Association and the American Academy of Pediatrics, but it is important to repeat that this book *does not* replace certification. We recommend that everyone seek training in these skills by certified instructors. This type of training, along with the advice in this book, could help save a child's life.

In the first section of this book, you will learn how to identify problems. In the second section, you will read, in detail, about how to perform cardiopulmonary resuscitation (CPR) and the relief-of-choking skills. You will also learn how to call for help. Knowing how to treat an emergency problem helps to sustain life, but survival also depends upon the ability to reach experts who can treat the injured child. These sections are placed first in the book so that you can find them easily in an emergency. Next, you will learn how to prevent and treat the problems that most commonly require cardio-pulmonary resuscitation. The final section contains lists and resource information that may help you.

The chapter about preventing and treating childhood emergencies contains information about identifying hazards and eliminating them or reducing their risk. Many people find it difficult to "babyproof" a home, day-care center, or school all at once. To help you begin, experts of the American Academy of Pediatrics recommend the following five steps as effective measures that can be taken to avoid injury to children.

FIVE IMPORTANT STEPS TO HELP PREVENT INJURY

1. **Use an approved car restraint device for children, starting at birth.**

2. **Install smoke detectors in the halls outside of bedrooms and other places where fires may start.**

3. **Turn down the hot-water heater to 120°F (49°C).**

4. **Install window and stairway guards and gates to prevent falls.**

5. **Keep two one-ounce (thirty-milliliter) bottles of syrup of ipecac per child in the house. Use only with the advice of experts at your local poison control center.**

While reading this book you will become aware of changes to be made to remove hazards in your home, day-care center, or school. We encourage you to make these changes and to practice the skills that have been introduced. Evaluate your environment from your children's perspective and keep in mind that they are continually growing and developing.

THE ABCS OF ASSESSMENT

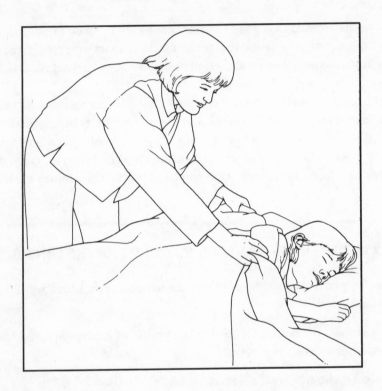

Assessment is a systematic way of observing a child to see if a problem exists. When observing a child, you assess:

1. Level of consciousness

2. *A*irway

3. *B*reathing

4. *C*irculation

5. Temperature

6. Hydration

The order in which you make these observations is extremely important. In any emergency situation, you assess the level of consciousness first because it will probably be the first change that you notice. Then, check that:

1. The child's *A*irway is open.

2. The child is *B*reathing.

3. The child's blood is *C*irculating.

The assessment of the **ABC**s is part of the cardiopulmonary resuscitation (CPR) sequence. If a child does not have an open Airway, is not Breathing, or does not have blood Circulating, then an emergency situation exists and someone must begin CPR immediately. This ABC assessment and CPR are more important than any other first-aid skills and should **always** be performed first.

Temperature and hydration are also important factors to assess in children because they can give helpful information about the cause or extent of the problem. They should be observed only *after* you have established an open Airway, Breathing, and Circulation.

In order to know if a child is in an emergency situation, it is important to know how the child behaves when he is well. The most accurate information is obtained when the child is calm and relaxed. Hold the child in your lap or have a familiar person distract the child while you perform the assessment. Use slow, deliberate motions and speak quietly and calmly.

LEVEL OF CONSCIOUSNESS

A person's level of consciousness is his alertness and awareness. The brain is responsible for the level of consciousness, which may be altered by infection, by injury, or by a problem with breathing or circulation that prevents oxygen from reaching the brain.

If a child is awake and in good health, he should respond in familiar ways to your voice and touch. If a child is asleep, he normally will respond to your voice and touch by moving or awakening. Make a note of the child's normal reaction upon being awakened

THE ABCS OF ASSESSMENT

from sleep and his normal movements, behavior, and temperament when awake.

A mild lack of oxygen may cause the child to be confused, restless, irritable, or weak. A severe lack of oxygen results in unconsciousness. Unconsciousness is a profound or deep state of unresponsiveness. It differs from sleep in that sleeping persons can be awakened whereas unconscious persons cannot be awakened.

The symptoms of unconsciousness are:

- Lack of spontaneous movement in response to shouts or stimulation
- Drooling
- Tongue fallen to back of the throat
- Eyes rolled back

In an emergency you should first determine the level of consciousness. Does the child respond when you gently shake him or shout his name? Does he respond when you flick his heels and lips? Can you detect an obvious change in his normal movements, behavior, or temperament? Does the child's behavior indicate confusion, restlessness, irritability, or weakness?

AIRWAY

How does a child's breathing work?

When a child breathes in, air travels down the airway to the lungs. The airway consists of the back of the throat, the trachea or windpipe, the epiglottis (a flap of tissue that closes over the trachea when you swallow so that food goes into the esophagus to the stomach and is not inhaled into the trachea), the bronchi, and finally the alveoli or air sacs of the lung. These air sacs are close to blood vessels, which take up the oxygen and carry it to the heart. The heart then pumps the oxygen through the arteries to the rest of the body.

An open airway is essential to allow oxygen to pass into the lungs and bloodstream. If any part of the airway becomes blocked because of improper positioning, an obstruction such as a piece of food (or other object), or swelling caused by infection, the child cannot get oxygen to the air sacs and to the blood. If oxygen cannot get to the blood, the brain and heart soon suffer. Ultimately, lack of oxygen can cause the heart to stop and brain damage to occur.

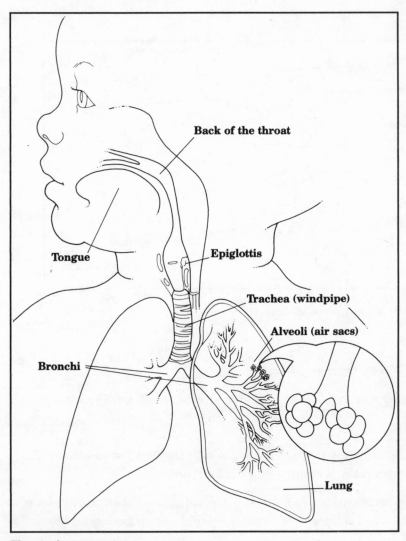

Back of the throat

Tongue

Epiglottis

Trachea (windpipe)

Alveoli (air sacs)

Bronchi

Lung

The respiratory system

THE ABCS OF ASSESSMENT

When assessing a child during an emergency, first note the level of consciousness. Then make sure that the airway is positioned so that it is open. Once you make sure that the airway is properly positioned, the next step is to make sure that the child is breathing on his own.

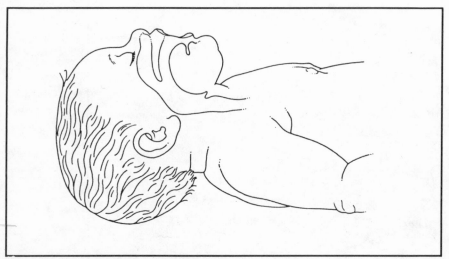

Proper position for open airway. Note that nose and ear are aligned perpendicular to floor.

BREATHING

Most childhood emergencies are the result of breathing problems. There are several reasons for this:

1. Babies breathe mainly through their noses for the first few months of life. A stuffy nose can make breathing difficult for them.

2. Swallowing and chewing are not well coordinated until about four years of age, so babies and children are more likely to choke on foods than are adults.

3. Infections of the sinuses, throat, and lungs are quite common in children. Since it takes them a few years to build immunity to bacteria and viruses in the environment, children are at high risk for acquiring infections.

4. Children are vulnerable to such things as drowning, choking on objects, and smoke inhalation, which directly affect breathing.

5. Most young children have strong, healthy hearts and good blood circulation, so they have little chance of having heart attacks. If their hearts stop, lack of oxygen resulting from breathing problems is usually the cause.

How can you determine if a child has a problem breathing?

Most newborn babies breathe about thirty to fifty times per minute. The rate decreases as the child grows, so a ten-year-old child may breathe about twenty times per minute.

NORMAL RANGES OF RESPIRATORY RATES

Newborns	30–50 breaths/minute
2 years	24–32 breaths/minute
10 years	20–26 breaths/minute
Adults	12–18 breaths/minute

Newborn babies do not breathe as regularly as adults, because the respiratory control center in the brain is still developing. They may breathe faster for a few seconds, more slowly for a few seconds, and then may stop temporarily.

Babies normally stop breathing temporarily for a few seconds, but if a baby does not breathe after ten to fifteen seconds, his condition is abnormal and is called *apnea*. Apnea is a failure to breathe that lasts longer than fifteen seconds. If you see this happening, start the CPR sequence immediately. (See page *24* for infants up to one year of age.)

It is important that you watch your child breathe when he is quiet or asleep so that you become comfortable counting respirations and know his normal respiratory rate or pattern. A breath in and out is counted as one breath.

> ### MY CHILD'S RESTING RATE
> ### OF BREATHING
>
> Newborn   _____breaths/minute
> 1–3 years   _____breaths/minute
> 3–5 years   _____breaths/minute
> 5–10 years _____breaths/minute

If a child shows any of the following signs of breathing difficulty, call your physician immediately. Start CPR sequence if the child is not breathing.

> ### CALL YOUR PHYSICIAN IF YOU OBSERVE ANY OF THE
> ### FOLLOWING. START CPR IF CHILD HAS STOPPED BREATHING.
>
> - **Rapid, slow, irregular, or absent breathing (if breathing is absent, start CPR sequence)**
> - **Blue-gray color inside the mouth (note: if this is accompanied by absent breathing, start CPR sequence)**
> - **Retractions (a pulling in of the muscles between ribs or below breastbone when working to breathe)**
> - **Flaring nostrils**
> - **Wheezing, grunting, or barking sound**
> - **Excessive sweating**
> - **Restless, agitated, irritable behavior**
> - **Weakness**
> - **Unconsciousness**

CIRCULATION

Circulation is the movement of blood through the heart and blood vessels. Circulation is dependent upon breathing. The drawing below shows how the two are related.

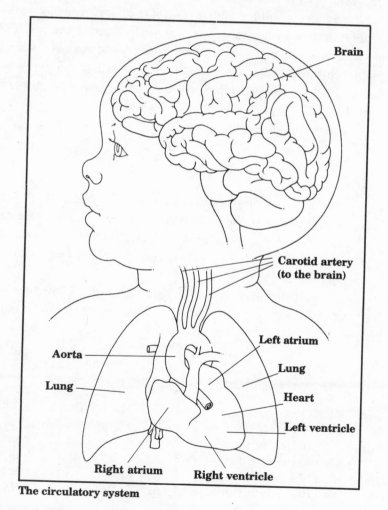

The circulatory system

The heart has four chambers. Blood from the body enters the heart in the *right atrium*. It is then pumped into the *right ventricle* and into the *pulmonary arteries*, which carry the blood to the blood vessels close to the air sacs of the lungs. At the level of the air sacs (alveoli), an exchange takes place. The blood gives up carbon dioxide to be expelled from the body as you breathe out and then picks up oxygen and carries it through the *pulmonary veins* into the *left atrium* of the heart. The blood passes into the *left ventricle* and into the *aorta*, where the oxygen-rich blood is pumped to the body.

The *carotid arteries* are two of the most important blood vessels, because they contain the oxygen-rich blood to be carried to the brain. When you perform cardiopulmonary resuscitation, you are providing just enough oxygen and pumping it to the brain and to the heart, the organs that need it the most.

Circulation is assessed by observing the pulse rate and tissue color.

PULSE

The pulse is a reflection of the heartbeat along the arteries and can be felt in different places on the body near the surface of the skin. The pulse rate can be determined by using a watch with a second hand and counting the number of beats in one minute. Use your index and middle fingers to check for a pulse. Do not use your thumb, which has its own pulse.

A normal pulse is regular and of moderate, equal strength. As you can see from the following chart, a baby's pulse is normally faster than that of a child or adult.

NORMAL RESTING HEART RATES	
Newborns	70–170 beats/minute
Age 1–2	80–130 beats/minute
Age 3–10	70–110 beats/minute
Adults	70–110 beats/minute

MY CHILD'S RESTING HEART RATES	
Newborn	_____beats/minute
Age 1–3	_____beats/minute
Age 3–5	_____beats/minute
Age 5–10	_____beats/minute

The normal pulse rate for a baby is anywhere between 70 and 170 beats per minute, depending upon the size of the baby, and decreases with age and increased size.

It is essential that you practice finding the child's normal pulse before a problem arises so that you are familiar with its location and quality. If the baby is less than one year of age, you should feel for a pulse at the brachial artery, located on the inside of the upper arm near the bone. Do not feel for a baby's pulse at the neck; a baby's airway is very flexible and pliable, and you might accidentally push too hard and cause an obstruction of the airway. The carotid pulse is also difficult to find in babies because of their fat, short necks.

If the child is older than one year of age, feel for a pulse at the carotid artery on one side of the neck next to the Adam's apple. Remember to use your index and middle fingers (not your thumb) to check the pulse.

When you feel for a pulse you should note if it is too fast, too slow, irregular, weak, or absent. A pulse that is too fast may be a sign of infection, bleeding, or shock. If you cannot feel a pulse, start CPR immediately.

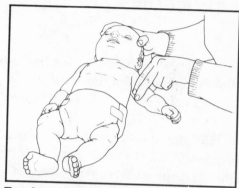

To take an infant's (age 0-1 year) pulse, use your fingertips to feel on the inside of the upper arm between the elbow and the shoulder.

To take a child's (age 1-8 years) pulse, place your fingertips on the child's Adam's apple, then slide your fingers into the groove next to the windpipe. Press gently and feel for the pulse of the carotid artery.

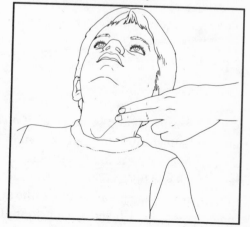

THE ABCS OF ASSESSMENT

SKIN COLOR

Like pulse, skin color is another indication of the adequacy of circulation. Observe the child at different times (at rest, at play, after eating) to become familiar with his normal range of color. Skin or tissue color that is different from normal may indicate a problem.

Pink skin color is considered normal and indicates that blood is receiving enough oxygen. Check the inside of the mouth for this color, since the oxygen-rich blood from the heart travels first to the head and brain. Because the tissues are inside the mouth, you should observe a pink color in a healthy person, regardless of complexion or race.

Red skin color may be normal if the child has been playing hard or is hot. It may also indicate a problem such as fever or carbon monoxide poisoning. Other terms used for red coloring are *flushed* and *cherry red*.

White skin color may be normal if the child is frightened, nervous, or feels faint. It may also indicate bleeding, shock, or low body temperature. The white colors can be described by the terms *pale, chalky,* or *waxen*.

Blue lips are normal if a child is cold. When this is the case, the inside of the mouth will still be pink. If the lips *and* the inside of the mouth are blue, ashen, gray, or dusky, the blood lacks oxygen. This is *not* normal, and you must begin the CPR sequence immediately.

TEMPERATURE

Temperature should be assessed if a child is warm and you think he is sick. An abnormal temperature may indicate an infection. Several methods and devices are available for measuring a child's temperature. Whichever one you choose, be consistent and note how it was taken. The age and condition of a child will help you determine whether to measure the temperature under the arm, orally, or rectally. Purchase the type of thermometer with which you are most familiar, be it Celsius (°C) or Fahrenheit (°F).

Two types of thermometers and three methods can be used to take a child's temperature. A rectal thermometer has a thick, rounded bulb to prevent injury to fragile rectal tissue. An oral thermometer has a pointed, long bulb. A rectal thermometer may be used to take rectal, axillary, or oral temperatures. An oral thermometer may be used to take only oral or axillary temperatures, because its pointed end might injure rectal tissue.

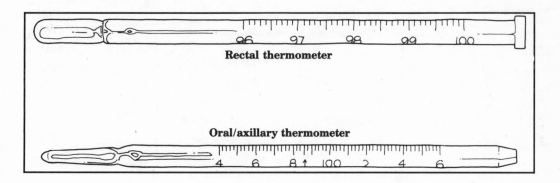

Rectal thermometer

Oral/axillary thermometer

1. *Axillary (Arm) Method.* This method is the safest method to use for young babies but can be used for persons of any age. Place the thermometer bulb under the armpit, and hold the arm close to the body for five minutes.

2. *Rectal Method.* Babies older than a few months and less than five years of age are candidates for rectal temperatures. Position an active child on his abdomen so you can lean on his body if necessary to prevent him from turning over. Lubricate the rectal thermometer with water-soluble jelly or petroleum jelly and insert it no more than one inch (two centimeters)—that is, the length of the mercury bulb. Keep the thermometer in place for two to five minutes.

3. *Oral Method.* Generally, a child older than five years of age can understand instructions to keep the thermometer beneath the tongue for at least five minutes. If the child is confused or uncooperative, select another method rather than risk the child biting, breaking, and swallowing the glass thermometer.

THE ABCS OF ASSESSMENT

Temperature variations above or below the average norms for age are not unusual in babies and children. Also, it is normal for there to be *less than* a one-degree (F) or one-half degree (C) difference in temperatures taken by different methods (see Average Normal Temperature chart below. Therefore, you must know your child's normal resting temperature before you can determine if he has a fever. A high temperature can be caused by time of day, clothing, activity, and environment but may indicate infection, dehydration, bleeding, or head injury. The following general guidelines will help to determine if fever is present.

**AVERAGE NORMAL
TEMPERATURES**

Celsius	37
Fahrenheit	98.6

A fever is a temperature over 38°C or 101°F by any temperature-taking method.

**MY CHILD'S RESTING
TEMPERATURES**

	Axillary	Oral	Rectal
Celsius	___	___	___
Fahrenheit	___	___	___

FEVER

A fever is a temperature greater than 101°F (38°C), by any temperature-taking method. Knowing when to call your physician is difficult because often children can have fevers when they are not very ill. Parents or caregivers want to be cautious and to obtain medical help if the child needs it, yet you do not want to bother your physician indiscriminately. The following guidelines may help you to decide when to call a physician.

GUIDELINES FOR PARENTS OF CHILD WITH FEVER
(Temperature Greater than 101°F or 38°C)

Call your doctor immediately if your child has a fever and:
- Is under two months of age
- The child's temperature is greater than 105°F (40.5°C)
- Your child is crying inconsolably
- Your child is difficult to awaken
- Your child is confused or delirious
- Your child has had a seizure
- Your child has a stiff neck
- Your child has purple spots on the skin
- Your child's breathing is labored, and he does not feel better after the nose is cleared
- Your child is acting very sick
- Your child has an underlying risk factor for serious infection (e.g., sickle-cell anemia)

Call your doctor during office hours if:
- Your child is 2–4 months old (unless fever is due to a DPT shot)
- Your child's temperature is between 104 and 105°F (40 and 40.5°C), especially if your child is under two years of age
- Burning or pain occurs with urination
- Fever has been present for more than 72 hours
- Fever has been present for more than 24 hours without an obvious cause or location of infection
- Fever went away for more than 24 hours and then returned
- Your child has a history of febrile seizures
- You have other questions

HYDRATION

Hydration is the amount of water in the body. It is important to assess hydration when a child is ill. The child who is sick, especially with fever or diarrhea, loses fluid quickly and can become dehydrated faster than an adult.

WARNING SIGNS OF DEHYDRATION

If you notice any of the following signs, you should contact your physician:
- Dry diapers for a longer period of time than normal, and darker, tea-colored urine with a strong odor
- Sunken eyes
- Dark circles under the eyes
- Skin that lacks its normal elastic quality when pinched and looks like the skin of an elderly person
- Dry mouth and tongue
- Absence of tears when the child cries
- Sunken fontanel, or soft spot, on the top of a baby's head
- Fast heart rate
- Weakness
- Unconsciousness

Remember, it is important to observe a child when there is no problem and to note what is normal for him in the areas of:

- General response or movement
- Rate of breathing
- Pulse rate
- Skin color
- Temperature
- Hydration

During an emergency, though, it is **most important** to assess the *ABC*s: *A*irway, *B*reathing, and *C*irculation. If any of these are abnormal, you must start CPR immediately.

PERFORMING THE ABCS OF CARDIOPULMONARY RESUSCITATION (CPR)

The heart of a healthy child is a wonderful pump and seldom fails to work. If it does fail, the cause is usually a breathing problem that prevents oxygen from reaching the heart. When you perform cardiopulmonary resuscitation (CPR) on a child who is not breathing or whose heart is not pumping, you are providing only enough blood and oxygen to supply the brain and the heart, so it is important to perform the skills correctly. No one is certain about how long children can live without oxygen before brain damage occurs. In adults brain damage can occur within four to six minutes. Cardiopulmonary resuscitation begun within minutes of an emergency's onset may increase the child's chance of survival.

In this chapter you will read about the skills that you should use to treat the most serious injuries, that is, those injuries that cause a child to have problems with **Airway**, **Breathing**, and **Circulation**. Throughout this book the importance of knowing and remembering the **ABC**s (**Airway**, **Breathing**, and **Circulation**) of cardiopulmonary resuscitation is stressed. This simple **ABC** memory device is used because it will help you to remember what to look for as well as how to treat the most serious problems. The **CPR** sequence comprises an entire set of skills, which includes assessing problems, calling for help, and administering treatment, including any or all of the **CPR** and relief-of-choking skills.

In many emergency situations, a child will sustain more than one injury, so you may have more than one problem to treat. By remembering the **ABC**s of **CPR**, you will know which problems to treat first. The other problems can wait until someone else arrives to help.

The **CPR** sequence is slightly different for an infant than for a child, and both will be described. Also, the relief-of-choking skills for the conscious and unconscious infant and child will be described. The relief-of-choking skills are actually part of cardiopulmonary resuscitation. They are skills to be used when someone has a problem with breathing because the airway is blocked. If you always think of the **ABC**s to help you find and resolve a problem, you will naturally use the proper skills at the appropriate time.

It is important to *practice* the skills presented in this chapter. We encourage you to attend a class in which *certified instructors* watch you practice on mannequins. You should *never* practice these skills on children. On page *129*, we provide tips and exercises to help you learn the steps of these skills. The skills presented in this book are based upon the 1986 standards of the American Heart Association.

OBTAINING HELP FROM THE EMERGENCY MEDICAL SYSTEM

It is very important to know how and when to obtain help if an emergency arises. Assessing the situation and performing CPR can often revive the child, but his chances of survival are improved if, in addition, the paramedics have been called and the victim is then brought to a hospital with an equipped emergency room and intensive-care services. Performing only cardiopulmonary resuscitation may not ultimately save the victim; you need expert medical assistance.

If an emergency arises, it is important to get help immediately. To save vital time in an emergency and to make obtaining help easier for caregivers, follow these five steps now to prepare for an emergency:

1. Post the following information by every telephone in case someone else is caring for the child at the time of the emergency:

>Your name
>Your address
>Your telephone number
>Nearest major cross streets or other nearby landmark.

PERFORMING THE ABCS OF CARDIOPULMONARY RESUSCITATION (CPR)

2. Post other important telephone numbers near the telephone:
   Poison control center
   Fire department
   Police department
   Family physician.
3. Notify authorities at the nearest fire and utilities departments if you have in the home a person with special problems, such as a disabled child, a baby with an apnea monitor, or anyone receiving oxygen or on a respirator.

4. Explain to non-English-speaking people and to children that in most areas of the United States, if they dial 911 and simply leave the telephone off the hook, the address will be displayed immediately on the dispatch computer. Policemen, firemen, and paramedics will be sent to that address.

5. In some communities in the United States, dialing 911 will not connect you with the emergency medical system. If the 911 number is not effective in your community, determine the fastest method for notifying those who provide emergency services.

DURING AN EMERGENCY, TAKE THE FOLLOWING STEPS

1. Dial 911.

2. Clearly state:
   Your name
   Your address
   Your telephone number
   Nearest major cross streets or other landmark
   A brief description of the problem.

3. Do not hang up until told to do so.

4. Open the front door (so that you will not have to leave the child again to open the door, the residence will be easily identifiable, and paramedics will not have to break the door down).

5. Try to remain calm and remember *A*irway, *B*reathing, and *C*irculation.

6. Continue to perform cardiopulmonary resuscitation until
   ■ help arrives *or*
   ■ the child is revived *or*
   ■ you are physically exhausted and cannot continue.

7. Do not take the child to the hospital. This will waste valuable time that you could use to perform cardiopulmonary resuscitation. Even if someone else can drive, you will not be able to perform cardiopulmonary resuscitation as effectively in a car and you may cause an accident because of your anxiety. Moreover, moving the child may cause additional injury.

CARDIOPULMONARY RESUSCITATION (CPR) FOR INFANTS (UNDER ONE YEAR)

SYMPTOMS

- Baby is not moving.
- Inside of baby's mouth may be blue.

TREATMENT

1. Establish unresponsiveness. You must determine whether the child is asleep or unconscious. You do not want to perform CPR if not necessary.

- Shake the baby gently.
- Flick the baby's heels.
- Shout the baby's name.

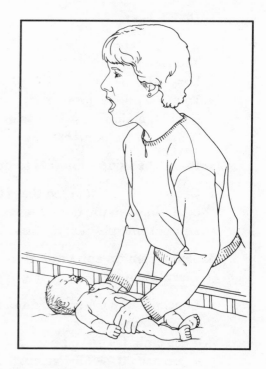

2. Call out for help.

- Even if you are alone, you should call for help because a neighbor or passerby may hear you.

3. Position the baby for CPR.

- Place the baby on his back on a hard surface, such as a table, counter, or uncarpeted floor. Pressing on the baby's chest (if necessary) makes the heart pump blood because you are squeezing it between the breastbone and a resistant surface.

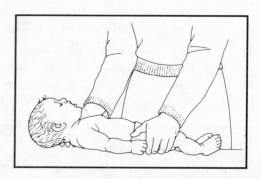

A I R W A Y

4. Open the airway.

- If no neck or back injury is suspected, tilt the head back until an imaginary line between the nose and ears is perpendicular to the floor.
- Do not hyperextend the baby's head and neck. This can close the airway or cause neck or back injury.
- If neck or back injury is suspected, try to use the "jaw-lift" technique. Place your thumb in the baby's mouth over the lower jaw and pull the jaw down toward the baby's feet and up away from the face to open the airway.

5. Once the *Airway* is open, continue on to *Breathing*.

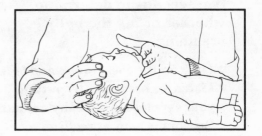

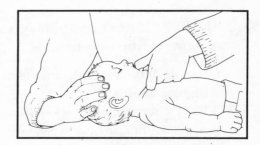

CARDIOPULMONARY RESUSCITATION (CPR) FOR INFANTS (UNDER ONE YEAR)

BREATHING

6. Look, listen, and feel for three to five seconds to determine whether or not the baby is breathing.

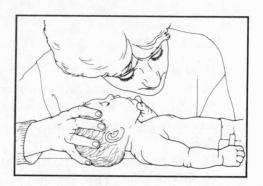

- Look for the chest to rise and fall.
- Listen for breathing by putting your ear close to the baby's mouth.
- Feel for the baby's breath on your cheek.
- Check the color of the inside of the mouth. Begin breathing for the baby if the inside of his mouth is blue. You must breathe for the baby to provide him with oxygen.

7. If the baby is not breathing, give two slow, gentle breaths.

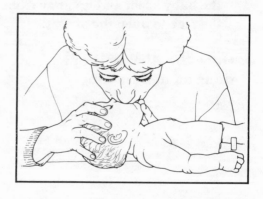

- Cover the baby's mouth and nose with your mouth.
- A baby's lung capacity is less than that of an adult, so give two small puffs of air as if you were blowing out a candle. Out of the corner of your eye, watch for the chest to rise.

8. If you cannot give two breaths because you meet resistance, call 911 and perform the relief-of-choking skill (see page 33, Choking Relief for Unconscious Infants).

9. After you are able to give two breaths, continue on to *Circulation*. You must check the circulation because, if the baby has not breathed for some time, his heart may have stopped.

CIRCULATION

10. Feel for a pulse for five to ten seconds.

- Feel for a brachial pulse in a baby on the inside of the upper arm between the elbow and the shoulder.

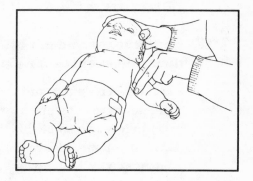

11. If you find no pulse and someone has come to help, have him dial 911.

- If there is a crowd of people, you must point to someone and say, "Go dial 911."
- If you are alone, continue CPR. You will dial 911 in one minute. It is important that a baby receive one minute of CPR without interruption — sometimes that is all that is necessary to revive a baby.

CARDIOPULMONARY RESUSCITATION (CPR) FOR INFANTS (UNDER ONE YEAR)

12. Begin compressions, five compressions to one breath.

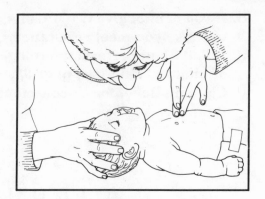

- Place your index finger on the breastbone between the nipples. Lift the index finger and use the middle and ring fingers to push down one-half to one inch (one to three centimeters), 100 times per minute. After every five compressions, give the baby a breath (count, "1, 2, 3, 4, 5 — BLOW — 1, 2, 3, 4, 5 — BLOW").

13. Continue for one minute and then stop to check for a pulse.

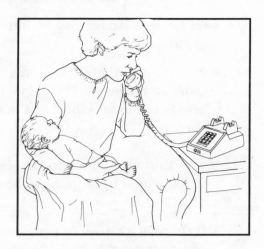

- If there is no pulse and if you did not have someone else call 911 before, do so at this time, even if you must leave the baby momentarily. If the telephone is far away, you may bring the baby with you.
- Give appropriate information.
- Do not hang up until told to do so.
- Open the front door.
- Return to the baby and check again for a pulse. If there is no pulse, continue breathing and compressions, stopping only to check for a pulse every five minutes.

- Continue until
  1. trained help arrives *or*
  2. the baby regains a pulse and respirations *or*
  3. you are physically unable to continue.

- If the pulse returns, reverse the ABCs sequence: check CBA. You know there is *C*irculation because you feel a pulse, so determine whether or not the baby is *B*reathing.

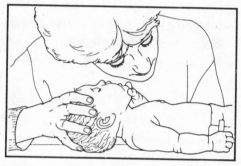

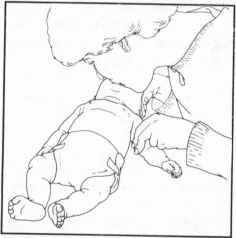

14. If the baby has a pulse but is not breathing, keep two fingers feeling the pulse and give breaths.
(Count aloud, "1, 2, 3, 4, 5 — BLOW — 1, 2, 3, 4, 5 — BLOW").

15. If the baby is breathing, continue backward through the ABCs (CBA). If the baby is still unconscious, you must keep the head properly positioned, keeping the *A*irway open. Babies' muscles relax when they are unconscious, and their airways can easily become blocked if they are not properly positioned.

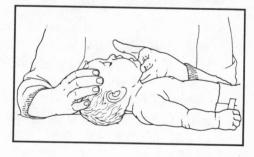

CHOKING RELIEF FOR CONSCIOUS INFANTS (UNDER ONE YEAR)

SYMPTOMS

- Baby is unable to make a sound. (You may hear only a high-pitched cry or ineffective cough.)
- Inside of the baby's mouth may be blue.

TREATMENT

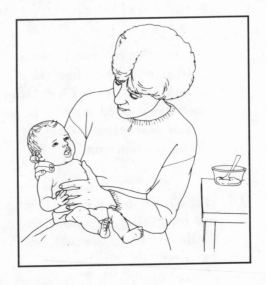

1. If the baby is coughing, *do nothing* except continue to observe. A cough is much more effective than any intervention. Intervention while a baby is coughing could cause a complete blockage of the airway.

IF THE BABY IS UNABLE TO CRY:

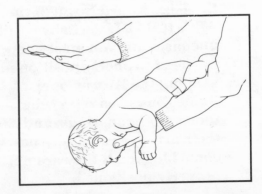

2. Give four back blows forcefully between the shoulder blades.

   - Support the baby's head, neck, and chest with one hand.
   - Hold the baby's head and body down at a sixty-degree angle.
   - Give four forceful blows between the shoulder blades with the heel of your other hand.

3. Give four chest thrusts.

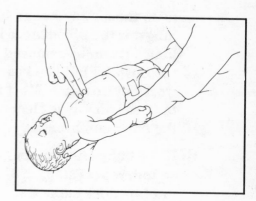

- Turn the baby over, keeping the head down at a sixty-degree angle.
- Place two fingers one finger-breadth below the nipple line on the breastbone to compress the chest one-half to one inch (one to three centimeters).
- You are pushing on the chest in the same way that you would if there were no pulse, but for a different reason. In this case, you are increasing the pressure on the airway to push out the object that is causing the baby to choke.

4. Keeping the baby's head down, lift the jaw and tongue with your thumb and remove the foreign object if you see it easily.

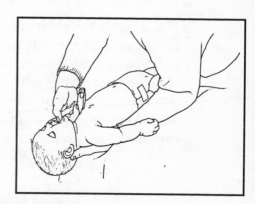

- Do not sweep the mouth blindly with your finger, or you may push the object down farther into the airway.

5. Observe the baby to determine if now he can make a sound. You may never see the object come up because it could be swallowed or it may be dislodged from the airway but go into the lungs. If the object goes into the lungs, it can be removed later at the hospital but is no cause for worry at this time. Most important, the airway is cleared and the baby can breathe.

6. If the baby still cannot make a sound, repeat steps 2, 3, 4, and 5 until he does make a sound or until he becomes unconscious. If the baby becomes unconscious, try to give two breaths, then call 911 and perform the relief-of-choking for unconscious infants. (See Choking Relief for Unconscious Infants, page 33.)

7. If the airway is cleared and the baby remains conscious, always call your physician, even if you cleared the airway with minimal intervention. He or she may wish to check that no parts of the object are in the lung.

In this relief-of-choking procedure, you are trying to dislodge the object from the small airways with back blows and then expel it with the chest thrusts. You do not perform the thrusts on the abdomen as you would for an older child because the muscles of babies are not developed enough to prevent injury.

CHOKING RELIEF FOR UNCONSCIOUS INFANTS (UNDER ONE YEAR)

SYMPTOMS

- The baby may be blue and not moving, but when you begin the ABCs of CPR you feel resistance when you try to give two breaths.
- A conscious, choking baby whom you are treating becomes blue and floppy.

TREATMENT

1. **Establish unresponsiveness.** Determine whether the baby is unconscious or asleep (you do not want to perform CPR if not necessary).
   - Shake the baby gently.
   - Flick the baby's heels.
   - Shout the baby's name.

2. **Call out for help.**
   - Even if you are alone, you should call for help because a neighbor or passerby may hear you.

3. **Position the baby.**
   - Place the baby on his back on a hard surface, such as a table, counter, or uncarpeted floor. Pressing on the baby's chest (if necessary) makes the heart pump blood because you are squeezing it between the breastbone and a resistant surface.

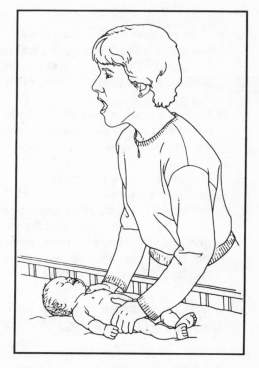

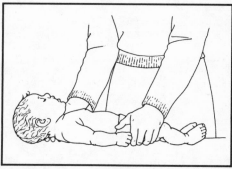

CHOKING RELIEF FOR UNCONSCIOUS INFANTS (UNDER ONE YEAR)

AIRWAY

4. Open the airway.

- If no neck or back injury is suspected, tilt the head back until an imaginary line between the nose and ears is perpendicular to the floor.
- Do not hyperextend the baby's head and neck. This can close the airway or cause neck or back injury.
- If neck or back injury is suspected, try to use the "jaw-lift" technique. Place your thumb in the baby's mouth over the lower jaw and pull the jaw down toward the baby's feet and up away from the face to open the airway.

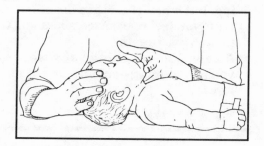

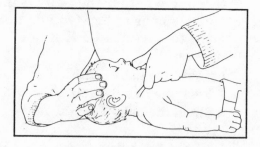

5. Once the *Airway* is open, continue on to *Breathing*.

BREATHING

6. Look, listen, and feel for three to five seconds to determine whether or not the baby is breathing.

- Look for the chest to rise and fall.
- Listen for breathing by putting your ear close to the baby's mouth.
- Feel for the baby's breath on your cheek.
- Check the color of the inside of the mouth. Attempt to begin breathing for the baby if the inside of the mouth is blue. You must try to breathe for the baby to provide him with oxygen.

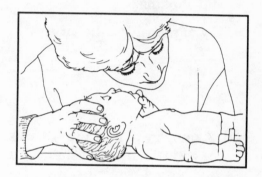

7. If the baby is not breathing, try to give two slow, gentle breaths.

- Cover the baby's mouth and nose with your mouth. Blow two small puffs of air, as if you were blowing out a candle. Out of the corner of your eye, watch for the chest to rise.

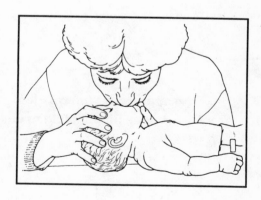

8. If you meet resistance when you blow or it feels as if you are blowing through a clogged straw, the airway is blocked and the baby is still choking.

9. Try to reposition the airway.

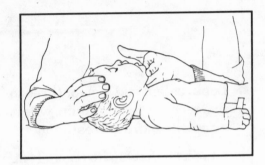

10. Again, try to give two breaths. If you *still* meet resistance, call 911, even if you must leave the baby momentarily. If the telephone is far away, you may bring the baby with you.

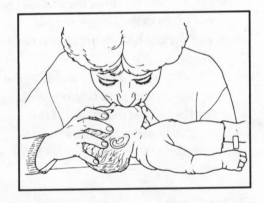

- Give appropriate information.
- Do not hang up until told to do so.
- Open the front door.

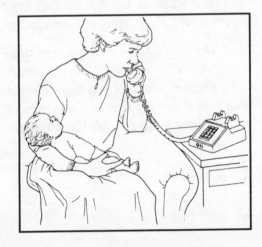

11. Give four back blows forcefully between the shoulder blades.

- Support the baby's head, neck, and chest with one hand.
- Hold the baby's head and body down at a sixty-degree angle.
- Give four forceful blows between the shoulder blades with the heel of your other hand.

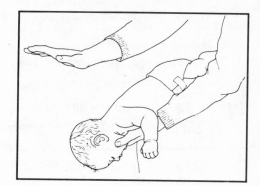

12. Give four chest thrusts.

- Turn the baby over, keeping the head down at a sixty-degree angle.
- Place two fingers one finger-breadth below the nipple line on the breastbone to compress the chest one-half to one inch (one to three centimeters).

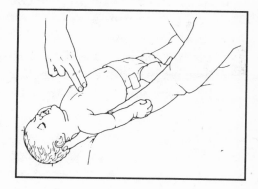

13. Keeping the baby's head down, lift the jaw and tongue with your thumb and remove the foreign object if you see it easily.

- Do not sweep the mouth blindly with your finger, or you may push the object down farther into the airway.

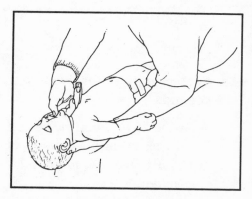

CHOKING RELIEF FOR UNCONSCIOUS INFANTS (UNDER ONE YEAR)

14. Try to give two breaths.

15. If you still meet resistance, re-position the airway and try again to give two breaths.

16. If you still meet resistance, re-peat steps 11, 12, and 13 (back blows, chest thrusts, and jaw lift) *until you are able to give two breaths.*

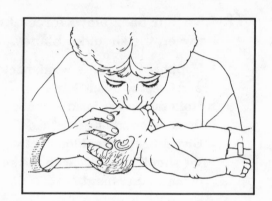

17. After you are able to give two breaths, continue on to *Circula-tion.* You must check the circulation because if the baby has not breathed for some time, his heart may have stopped.

CIRCULATION

18. Feel for a pulse for five to ten seconds.

- Feel for a brachial pulse in a baby on the inside of the upper arm between the elbow and the shoulder.

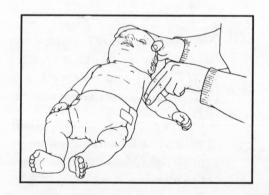

19. If you find no pulse, begin cardiac compressions and breaths, five compressions to one breath.

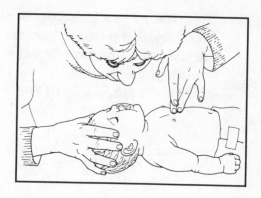

- Place your index finger on the breastbone between the nipples and use your middle and ring fingers to push down one-half to one inch, 100 times per minute. After every five compressions, give the baby a breath. (Count, "1, 2, 3, 4, 5 — BLOW — 1, 2, 3, 4, 5 — BLOW").

20. Continue for one minute and then stop to check for a pulse.

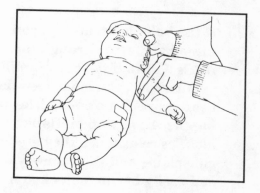

- If there is no pulse, continue breathing and compressions, stopping only to check for a pulse every five minutes.
- Continue to give CPR without stopping until trained help arrives *or* the child regains a pulse and breathes *or* you are physically unable to continue.

21. If the pulse returns, reverse ABC sequence: check CBA. You know there is *C*irculation because you feel a pulse, so determine if the baby is *B*reathing.

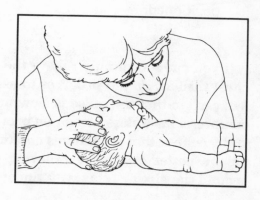

22. If the baby has a pulse but is not breathing, keep two fingers feeling the pulse and give breaths (count aloud, "1, 2, 3, 4, 5 — BLOW — 1, 2, 3, 4, 5 — BLOW").

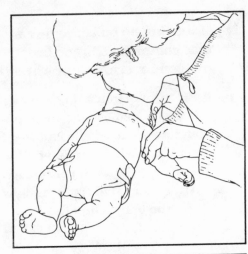

23. If the baby is breathing, continue backward through the ABCs (CBA). If the baby is still unconscious, you must keep the head properly positioned, keeping the Airway open. Babies' muscles relax when they are unconscious, and their airways can easily become blocked if they are not properly positioned.

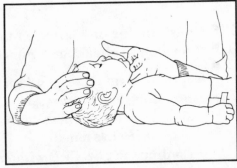

If you cannot initially relieve the obstruction with the back blows and chest thrusts, *do not* progress to assess and treat *Circulation*, even if you feel certain that the pulse is slowing. The baby cannot benefit from chest compressions unless he can be provided with oxygen from your breaths.

Remember that if a baby is choking and becomes unconscious, you will have a better chance of relieving the obstruction because the muscles around the airway relax with unconsciousness.

SYMPTOMS

- Child is not moving.
- Inside of child's mouth may be blue.

TREATMENT

1. Establish unresponsiveness. You must determine whether the child is asleep or unconscious. You do not want to perform CPR if not necessary.

- Shake the child gently.
- Flick the child's heels.
- Shout the child's name.

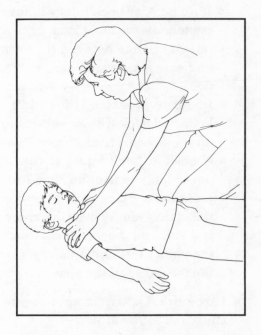

2. Call out for help.

- Even if you are alone, you should call for help because a neighbor or passerby may hear you.

3. Position the child.

- Place the child on his back on a hard surface, such as a table, counter, or uncarpeted floor. Pressing on the child's chest (if necessary) makes the heart pump blood because you are squeezing it between the breastbone and a resistant surface.

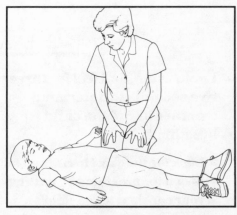

CARDIOPULMONARY RESUSCITATION FOR CHILDREN (ONE TO EIGHT YEARS)

A I R W A Y

4. **Open the airway.**

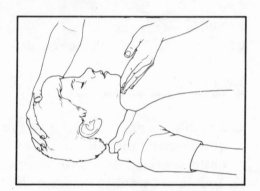

- **If no neck or back injury is suspected, tilt the head back until an imaginary line between the nose and ears is perpendicular to the floor.**
- **Do not hyperextend the child's head and neck. This can close the airway or cause neck or back injury.**
- **If neck or back injury is suspected, try to use the "jaw-lift" technique. Place your thumb in the child's mouth over the lower jaw and pull the jaw down toward the child's feet and up away from the face to open the airway.**

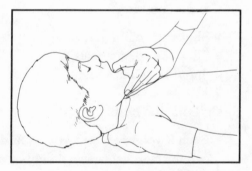

5. **Once the *Airway* is open, continue on to *Breathing*.**

B R E A T H I N G

6. **Look, listen, and feel for three to five seconds to determine whether or not the child is breathing.**

- **Look for the chest to rise and fall.**
- **Listen for breathing by putting your ear close to the child's mouth.**

- Feel for the child's breath on your cheek.
- Check the color of the inside of the mouth. Begin breathing for the child if the inside of his mouth is blue. You must breathe for the child to provide him with oxygen.

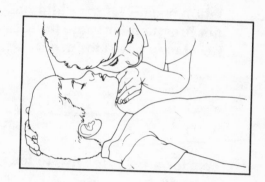

7. If the child is not breathing, give two slow, gentle breaths.

- Pinch the child's nose shut and cover his mouth with your mouth to form an airtight seal.
- A child's lung capacity is less than that of an adult, so give two small puffs of air as if you were blowing out a candle. Out of the corner of your eye, watch for the chest to rise.

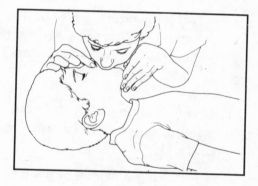

8. If you cannot give two breaths because you meet resistance, call 911 and perform the relief-of-choking skill (see page *50*, Choking Relief for Unconscious Children).

9. After you are able to give two breaths, continue on to *Circulation*. You must check the circu-

lation because if the child has not breathed for some time, his heart may have stopped.

C I R C U L A T I O N

10. Feel for a pulse for five to ten seconds.

   ■ Feel for a carotid pulse in the neck by sliding two fingers onto the groove next to the Adam's apple.

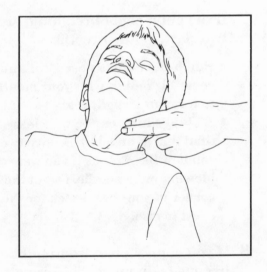

11. If you find no pulse and someone has come to help, have him dial 911.

   ■ If there is a crowd of people, you must point to someone and say, "Go dial 911."
   ■ If you are alone, continue CPR. You will dial 911 in one minute. It is important that a child receive one minute of CPR without interruption — sometimes that is all that is necessary to revive the child.

12. Begin compressions, five compressions to one breath.

- Place the heel of one hand two finger-breadths above where the ribs meet on the breastbone. Push down one to one and one-half inches (two to four centimeters), 100 times per minute. After every five compressions, give the child a breath (count, "1, 2, 3, 4, 5 — BLOW — 1, 2, 3, 4, 5 — BLOW").

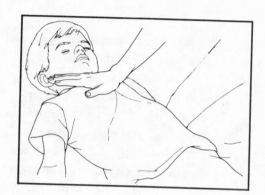

13. Continue for one minute and then stop to check for a pulse.

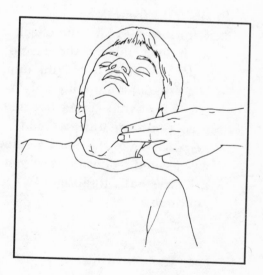

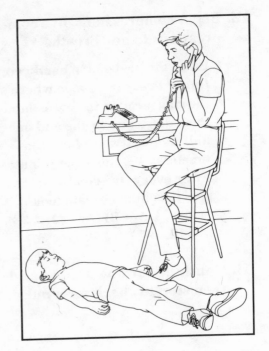

- If there is no pulse and you did not have someone else call 911 before, do so at this time, even if you must leave the child momentarily. If the telephone is far away and you can lift the child, bring him with you, but do not try this if it might waste time or the child has other injuries.
- Give appropriate information.
- Do not hang up until told to do so.
- Open the front door.
- Return to the child and check again for a pulse. If there is no pulse, continue breathing and compressions, stopping only to check for a pulse every five minutes. Continue until trained help arrives *or* the child regains a pulse and respirations *or* you are physically unable to continue.

■ If the pulse returns, reverse the ABC sequence: check CBA. You know there is *C*irculation because you feel a pulse, so determine whether or not the child is *B*reathing.

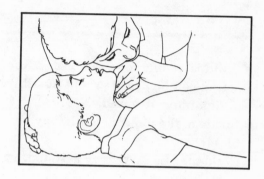

14. If the child has a pulse but is not breathing, keep two fingers feeling the pulse and give breaths (count "1, 2, 3, 4, 5 — BLOW — 1, 2, 3, 4, 5 — BLOW").

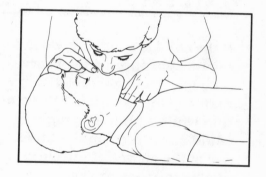

15. If the child is breathing, continue backward through the ABCs (CBA). If the child is still unconscious, you must keep the head properly positioned, keeping the *A*irway open. Children's muscles relax when they are unconscious, and their airways can easily become blocked if they are not properly positioned.

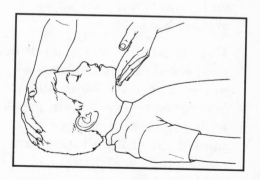

CHOKING RELIEF FOR CONSCIOUS CHILDREN (ONE TO EIGHT YEARS)

SYMPTOMS

- Child is unable to speak or cry. No sound can be heard except possibly a high-pitched sound.
- Inside of the child's mouth may be blue.
- Child may be extremely agitated.

TREATMENT

1. If the child is coughing, *do nothing* except continue to observe. A cough is much more effective than any intervention. Intervention while a child is coughing could cause a complete blockage of the airway. If the child is unable to speak or cry:

2. Stand, kneel, or sit behind the child and wrap your arms around his waist.

3. Make a fist with one hand. Place your hand on the child's abdomen above the belly button and below where the ribs meet, with your thumb turned in toward the child. Place your other hand over the fist.

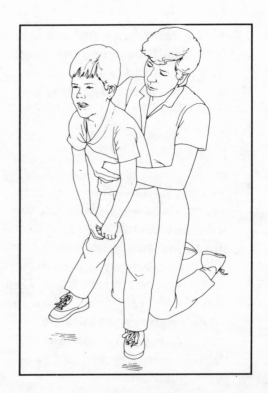

4. Press your hands into the abdomen with gentle, quick, upward thrusts until the child is able to make a sound or becomes unconscious. You may never see the object come up because it could be swallowed or it may be dislodged from the airway but go into the lungs. If the object goes into the lungs, it can be removed later at the hospital but is no cause for worry at this time. Most important, the airway is cleared and the child can breathe. If the child becomes unconscious, try to give two breaths and call 911 (See Choking Relief for Unconscious Children, page *50*).

5. If the airway is cleared and the child remains conscious, always call your physician, even if the child seems fine. He or she may want to check that no parts of the object are in the lung.

CHOKING RELIEF FOR UNCONSCIOUS CHILDREN (ONE TO EIGHT YEARS)

SYMPTOMS

- The child may be blue and not moving, but when you begin the ABCs of CPR you feel resistance when you try to give two breaths.
- A conscious, choking child whom you are treating becomes blue and floppy.

TREATMENT

1. **Establish unresponsiveness.** You must determine whether the child is unconscious or asleep. You do not want to perform CPR if not necessary.

   - Shake the child gently.
   - Flick the child's heels.
   - Shout the child's name.

2. **Call out for help.**

   - Even if you are alone, you should call for help because a neighbor or passerby may hear you.

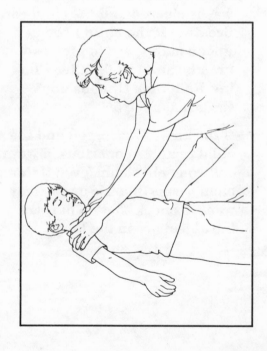

CHOKING RELIEF FOR UNCONSCIOUS CHILDREN (ONE TO EIGHT YEARS)

B R E A T H I N G

6. Look, listen, and feel for three to five seconds to determine whether or not the child is breathing.

- Look for the chest to rise and fall.
- Listen for breathing by putting your ear close to the child's mouth.
- Feel for the child's breath on your cheek.
- Check the color of the inside of the mouth. Attempt to begin breathing for the child if the inside of the mouth is blue. You must try to breathe for the child to provide him with oxygen.

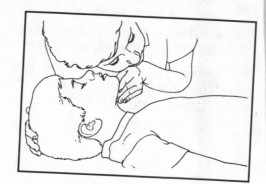

7. If the child is not breathing, try to give two slow, gentle breaths.

- Pinch the child's nose shut and cover his mouth with your mouth to form an airtight seal.
- Blow two puffs into the child's mouth as if you were blowing out a candle. Out of the corner of your eye, watch for the chest to rise.

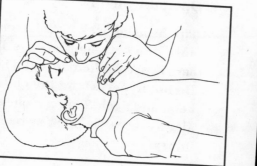
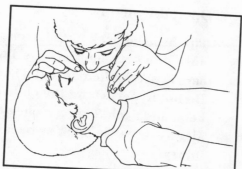

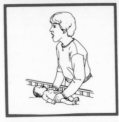

Shake baby and shout his name.

Call out for help.

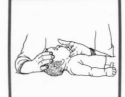

1. Open AIRWAY by tilting the head back slightly.

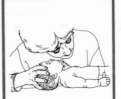

2. Look, listen, and feel to determine if baby is BREATHING.

If baby _is_ breathing, maintain Airway (step #1).

If baby _is not_ breathing…

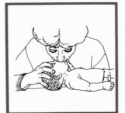

Cover the baby's nose and mouth with your mouth and give two slow, gentle puffs of air.

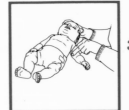

3. Check CIRCULATION.
Feel for brachial (upper arm) pulse.

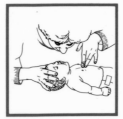

If you do not feel a pulse, place two fingers just below nipple line on the breastbone and push five times, then give one breath. Count as you push, "1, 2, 3, 4, 5—BLOW—1, 2, 3, 4, 5—BLOW," for one minute, then check again for pulse. Call 911 if it has not been done already. If there is no pulse, continue breathing and compressions, stopping only every five minutes to check for pulse. When you feel pulse, check Breathing (step #2). When baby has a pulse and is breathing, maintain Airway (step #1).

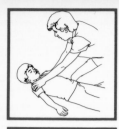

Shake child and shout his name.

Call out for help.

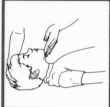

1. Open AIRWAY by tilting the head back slightly.

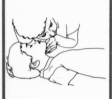

2. Look, listen, and feel to determine if child is BREATHING.

If child is breathing, maintain Airway (step #1).

If child is not breathing...

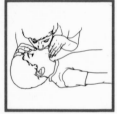

Pinch the child's nose and give two slow, gentle puffs of air.

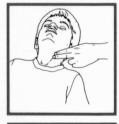

3. Check CIRCULATION.
    Feel for carotid (neck) pulse.

If you do not feel a pulse, place heel of hand two finger-breadths above where ribs meet on breastbone and push five times, then give one breath. Count as you push, "1, 2, 3, 4, 5—BLOW—1, 2, 3, 4, 5—BLOW," for one minute, then check again for pulse. Call 911 if it has not been done already. If there is no pulse, continue breathing and compressions, stopping only every five minutes to check for pulse. When you feel pulse, check Breathing (step #2). When child has a pulse and is breathing, maintain Airway (step #1).

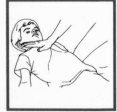

CHOKING RELIEF FOR UNC
CHILDREN (ONE TO EIGHT

3. Position the child.

■ Place the child on his back on a hard surface, such as a table, counter, or uncarpeted floor. Pressing on the child's chest (if necessary) makes the heart pump blood because you are squeezing it between the breastbone and a resistant surface.

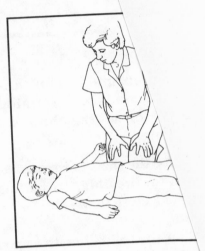

A I R W A Y

4. Open the airway.

■ Tip the head back until an imaginary line between the nose and ears is perpendicular to the floor.
■ Do not hyperextend the child's head and neck. This can close the airway or cause neck or back injury.

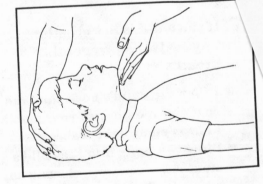

5. Once the *Airway* is open, continue on to *Breathing*.

8. If you meet resistance when you blow or it feels as if you are blowing through a clogged straw, the airway is blocked and the child is still choking.

9. Try to reposition the airway.

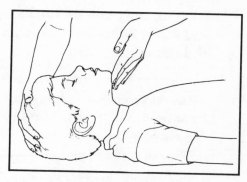

10. Again, try to give two breaths. If you *still* meet resistance, call 911, even if you must leave the child momentarily.

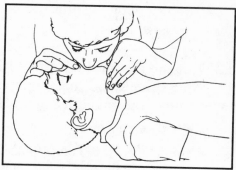

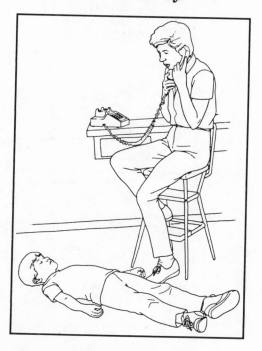

- Give appropriate information.
- Do not hang up until told to do so.
- Open the front door.

11. Position the child on his back and kneel at his feet. Give six abdominal thrusts.

- Place the heel of one hand midline on the child's abdomen, above the belly button and below where the ribs meet.
- Place the other hand on top of the first and press into the abdomen with a gentle, quick upward thrust.

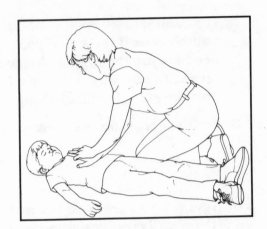

12. Lift the jaw and tongue with your thumb and forefinger and remove the foreign object if you see it easily.

- Do not sweep the mouth blindly with your finger, or you may push the object down farther into the airway.

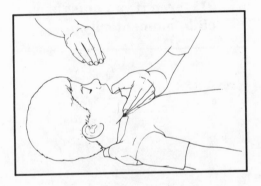

13. Try to give two breaths.

14. If you still meet resistance, reposition the airway and try again to give two breaths.

15. If you still meet resistance, repeat steps 11 and 12 (abdominal thrusts and jaw lift) *until you are able to give two breaths.*

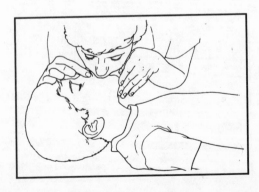

16. After you are able to give two breaths, continue on to *Circulation.* You must check the circulation because if the child has not breathed for some time, his heart may have stopped.

CIRCULATION

17. Feel for a pulse for five to ten seconds.

- Feel for a carotid pulse in the neck by sliding two fingers into the groove next to the Adam's apple.

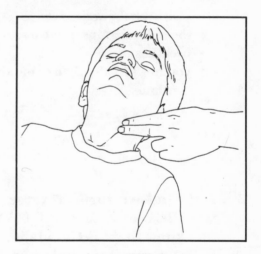

18. If you find no pulse, begin cardiac compressions and breaths, five compressions to one breath.

- Place the heel of one hand two finger-breadths above where the ribs meet on the breastbone. Push down one to one and one-half inches (two to four centimeters), 100 times per minute. After every five compressions, give the child a breath (count, "1, 2, 3, 4, 5 — BLOW — 1, 2, 3, 4, 5 — BLOW").

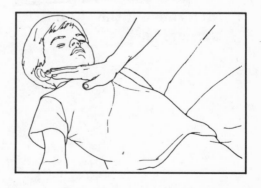

CHOKING RELIEF FOR UNCONSCIOUS CHILDREN (ONE TO EIGHT YEARS)

19. Continue for one minute and then stop to check for a pulse.

- If there is no pulse, continue breathing and compressions, stopping only to check for a pulse every five minutes.
- Continue to give CPR without stopping until

1. trained help arrives *or*
2. the child regains a pulse and breathes *or*
3. you are physically unable to continue.

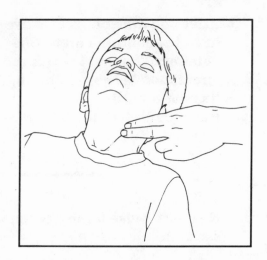

20. If the pulse returns, reverse the ABC sequence: check CBA. You know there is *C*irculation because you feel a pulse, so determine if the child is *B*reathing.

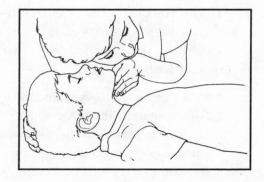

21. If the child has a pulse but is not breathing, keep two fingers feeling the pulse and give breaths (count "1, 2, 3, 4, 5 — BLOW — 1, 2, 3, 4, 5 — BLOW").

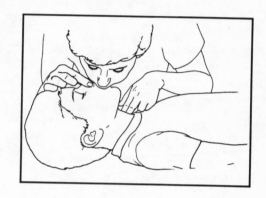

22. If the child is breathing, continue backward through the ABCs (CBA). If the child is still unconscious, you must keep the head properly positioned, keeping the *Airway* open. Children's muscles relax when they are unconscious, and their airways can easily become blocked if they are not properly positioned.

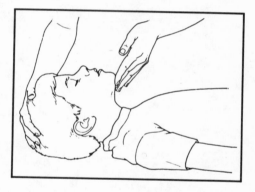

If you cannot initially relieve the obstruction with the abdominal thrusts, *do not* progress to assess and treat *C*irculation, even if you feel certain that the pulse is slowing. The child cannot benefit from chest compressions unless he can be provided with oxygen from your breaths.

Remember that if a child is choking and becomes unconscious, you will have a better chance of relieving the obstruction because the muscles around the airway relax with unconsciousness.

CARDIOPULMONARY RESUSCITATION (CPR) SUMMARY

The CPR and relief-of-choking sequences can seem overwhelming, but they are really very logical if you remember *A-B-C*, where *A* is *Air*way, *B* is *B*reathing, and *C* is *C*irculation. By assessing and treating the infant or child according to the ABCs of CPR, you may improve his chance of survival.

Here are five other points to remember:

1. The relief-of-choking skills are part of the ABCs of the CPR sequence. They are skills that you use when you cannot treat beyond *Airway* because it is blocked.
2. Continue to aid a *conscious* choking baby or child until he can make a sound.
3. Continue to aid an *unconscious* choking baby or child until you are able to give two breaths through the airway, then check circulation.
4. Once you establish that the child has an open airway, is breathing, and has circulation, do not leave the child until you assess and treat the ABCs, backward. If the child has a pulse, you must check that he is breathing. If he is not breathing, then you breathe for him. If he is breathing, then you check the airway and hold it open until he regains consciousness. You must assess and treat the ABCs and then the CBAs of cardiopulmonary resuscitation.
5. You should practice these skills on mannequins under the supervision of *certified instructors*. You should *never* practice on children.

PREVENTION AND TREATMENT
OF COMMON CHILDHOOD EMERGENCIES

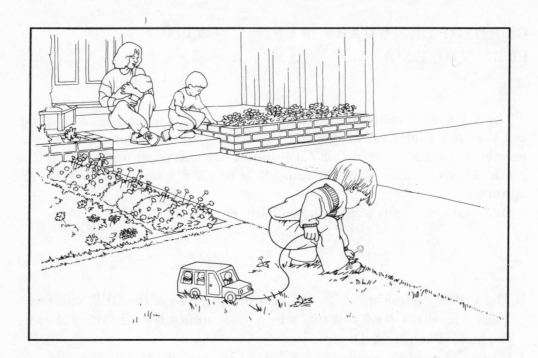

Any childhood emergency is stressful and sometimes tragic for the person caring for that child. Knowing beforehand what emergency measures to perform, including cardiopulmonary resuscitation (CPR), can give you a sense of confidence and security, but it is always better to try to *prevent* emergency situations.

In this chapter we present the leading causes of childhood emergencies, as identified by members of the American Academy of Pediatrics. In each case we outline ways to *prevent* an emergency situation from Occurring, followed by a description of the proper *treatment*, should injury or illness take place. The emergencies considered are:

- Automobile accidents
- Bleeding
- Burns
- Choking
- Drowning

- Electric shock
- Head, neck, and back injuries
- Infections of the upper airway
- Infectious disease in day-care centers and schools
- Injuries: miscellaneous
- Poisoning
- Seizures caused by fever
- Smoke inhalation
- Sudden infant death syndrome (SIDS)(cannot be prevented)

After you read this chapter and are ready to childproof your home, day-care center, or school, remember that it is best to look at your environment from the child's perspective. This may include kneeling on the floor and looking at the room from the child's eye level to see what items might be interesting but hazardous. Set aside some time each day to childproof your home, day-care center, or school in one or two of the areas identified. You can use the suggestions under the "Prevention" headings in the following pages. Children are always growing and developing new skills, so prevention is a continual process. You cannot complete it in a day!

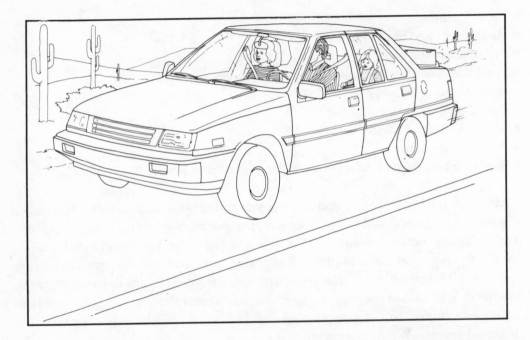

Automobile accidents are the primary cause of death and disability among children under the age of four and account for almost 25 percent of all accidental deaths of children aged one to fourteen. Most of these injuries happen to children who are not in car seats or proper restraint devices or who are not wearing seat belts. Holding a child in your arms is not sufficient protection and could lead to the child being crushed between you and the dashboard or being thrown around or from the car. Car safety begins on the day you bring your baby home from the hospital. If a child always uses a car seat or restraint, he will know no other way of riding in a car and will probably not fuss or complain.

PREVENTION

- Do not use infant seats or car beds as a substitute for a car seat.
- Be a defensive, cautious driver. Observe all car and highway rules and speed limits.

- Make sure that your car is well maintained and that brakes, tires, steering, windshield wipers, lights, signals, and horn work properly.
- Wear your seat belt as an example for the child and to protect yourself.
- Always use a car seat that meets or exceeds government safety standards. Different styles are available for different ages and weights, so make sure to get the appropriate model for your child and switch to a new model when the old one is outgrown. If you cannot afford a car seat, inquire about rental or used car seats from your local office of the National Highway Traffic Safety Administration, from the American Automobile Association, or from another community group. To receive a free pamphlet, contact the National Highway Traffic Safety Administration (see Resources, page *140,* for telephone number).

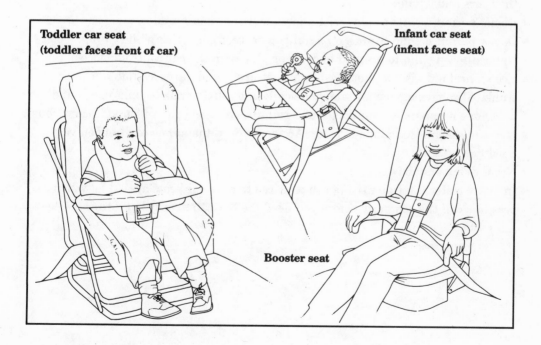

Toddler car seat (toddler faces front of car)

Infant car seat (infant faces seat)

Booster seat

AUTOMOBILE ACCIDENTS

- Always use the car seat correctly and know how to install it properly before you buy it.
- The safest location for a car seat is in the center of the rear seat.
- Face children weighing up to twenty pounds (nine kilograms) backward. Their backs withstand impact better than their abdomens because they do not have much abdominal muscle development at a young age.
- If, for some reason beyond your control, you do not have a car seat, the safest place for the baby or child is on the floor in the back seat.
- Use a car seat until the child is four years old or weighs forty pounds (eighteen kilograms). Then use a booster seat and seat belt until the child is big enough to have the belt rest on his pelvis, *not* his abdomen, which still cannot sustain an impact without possible injury.
- Make sure that your child's fingers, arms, and legs are safely inside before closing the doors and windows.
- Do not permit a child to play with the windows or door handles.
- Do not permit a child to suck on a lollipop or ice-cream stick while riding.
- Never allow a child to pretend to drive or play with the car control devices.
- Keep a first-aid kit, blanket, flashlight, batteries, and flares available in your trunk. Also have money for telephone calls and a list of names, addresses, and telephone numbers of your doctor and relatives in case you are found unconscious.
- Never leave children alone in a car. Accidents or kidnappings can happen very quickly.
- Never drink and drive.
- In many states, taxicab drivers are required to have car seats available. When possible, call the company before you need the taxicab to ask that a car seat be available.

TREATMENT

1. Assess *A*irway, *B*reathing, and *C*irculation, and start CPR if necessary. (See page *24* for infants under one year of age; see page *41* for children aged one to eight.)

2. Always assume that there may be a head, neck, or back injury. If CPR is necessary, try to use the jaw-lift technique to deliver breaths (see page *25*).

3. *Do not* move the child unless it is absolutely necessary, that is, if the area is dangerous (for example, if the child is in the middle of traffic, if you think that the car's gas tank may explode, or if CPR is necessary). When moving an accident victim, avoid twisting the neck or spine. Move him as a single unit, keeping the head in line with the spinal column.

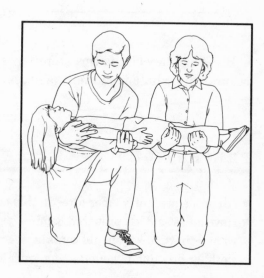

4. Treat for bleeding and shock.

BLEEDING

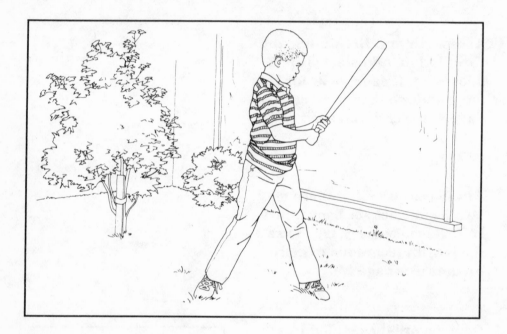

Bleeding may be life threatening, especially if an artery has been cut. If this occurs, immediate treatment is necessary.

PREVENTION

- All of the preventive measures in this book could prevent bleeding.
- Have a first-aid kit prepared before a problem arises. (For a complete description of what a first-aid kit should contain, see page *130*.) It should include gauze or sterile cloth for dressing a wound and a tourniquet (a long, thin strip of material).

■ Practice finding pressure points on your child. Pressure points are areas on the body where you feel pulses. These can be pressed firmly to stop serious bleeding. Some easily found pressure points are noted in this diagram:

SYMPTOMS OF BLEEDING

■ Excessive loss of blood can cause shock. Be aware of the signs of shock:

> Rapid, weak pulse
> Irregular breathing
> Nausea and vomiting
> Thirst
> Pale, moist, blotchy skin
> Mental confusion
> Anxiety
> Weakness
> Unconsciousness

■ Be aware of the signs of external bleeding:

> Open, visible wound
> Bleeding from artery: spurting, bright red blood
> Bleeding from vein: continuous flow of dark, red blood
> Signs of shock

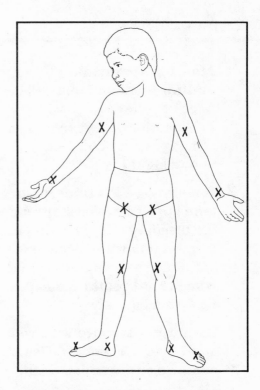

■ Be aware of the signs of internal bleeding:

> Perhaps no visible wound
> Bruised skin, indicating a blow or hard impact to the body
> Hard abdomen
> Swelling
> Bloody or dark brown vomit or stool, indicating old blood
> Signs of shock

BLEEDING

TREATMENT

1. Monitor *A*irway, *B*reathing, and *C*irculation. Start CPR if necessary. (See page *24* for infants under one year of age; see page *41* for children aged one to eight.)

2. Performing CPR (if necessary) takes priority over stopping the bleeding. The bleeding may stop on its own or someone may come to help, but a child who is not breathing needs CPR immediately.

3. Use direct pressure with your hand over the wound. Use a bandage or any clean cloth.

4. Elevate the wounded body part above the level of the heart.

5. Apply firm pressure, using a sterile or clean piece of gauze or cloth. Do not remove it to check if the bleeding has stopped, as this will disrupt the clot and cause bleeding to continue. If the dressing becomes soaked, apply another one on top of it.

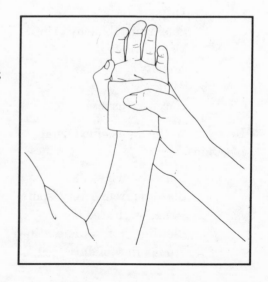

6. If bleeding continues, apply pressure to the artery where you feel a pulse (above the cut) between the cut and the heart. This is a pressure point. Use only enough pressure to stop the bleeding without stopping the circulation. Check fingers or toes to make sure that circulation continues below the place where you have applied pressure. Pink or blue skin below the pressure point means that circulation is present even if it is slowed. White skin means there is *no* circulation to the area. If you see white skin, release the pressure *immediately* until the skin becomes blue or pink. If the cut is on the head, apply pressure directly to the cut. *Do not* apply pressure to the pulse in the neck, or you may stop all circulation to the head and brain.

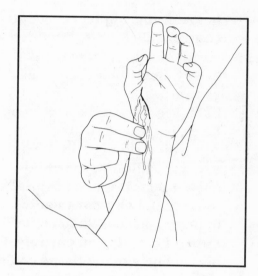

7. A tourniquet is a long, thin strip of material that is tied just above the spurting blood between a cut artery and the heart. A tourniquet is used to control only severe, life-threatening bleeding from a cut artery. Items that can be used as tourniquets include panty hose, scarves, thin socks, shoe laces, belts, or any long, narrow, soft strip of cloth. If you use a tourniquet, the child should be taken to a hospital immediately by paramedics (call 911), because a tourniquet cuts off circulation entirely and damage to the tissue could soon occur. You do not want to cut off any more circulation than necessary to the rest of the limb. A tourniquet should be tied around the limb, finger, or toe (never around the neck or torso), and the ends of it should be twisted until the spurting stops. Note the exact time that you apply the tourniquet, and release the pressure every few minutes. Release pressure immediately if you see that the extremity has turned white. If spurting blood continues, tighten the tourniquet and repeat the process.

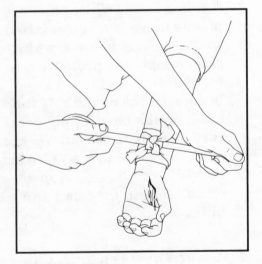

8. If a body part has been severed, wrap the severed part in cool, moist bandages or clean cloth and place it in a plastic bag that can be placed on ice. Never put the severed part *directly* on ice, or the tissue may be damaged.

9. Do not remove punctured or impaled objects. If the child must be moved, do so gently, then treat for bleeding and shock.

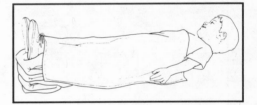

10. Treat for shock by elevating the legs, if possible, and covering the child with a blanket or clothes.

11. To stop a nosebleed, apply direct pressure by firmly pinching both nostrils with a thumb and forefinger. The child should sit down and lean slightly forward (not backward: blood will run down the throat and the child might inhale it).

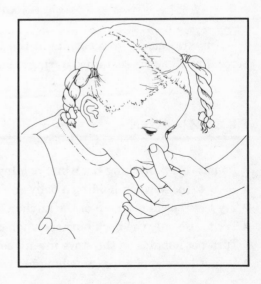

BURNS

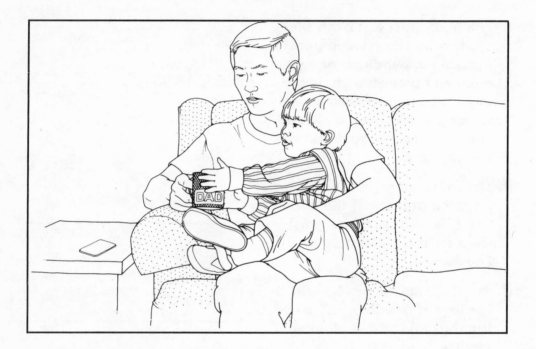

Burns are caused by accidents in the home as well as by fires. Approximately 90 percent of all burns sustained during infancy are caused by scalding.

PREVENTION

- Do not carry anything hot while holding a baby or child.
- Do not smoke when holding a baby or child.
- Try to keep children out of the kitchen while you are cooking.
- Try to use only the back burners when cooking.
- Turn pot handles on the stove inward so that toddlers cannot grab and pull them.
- Do not leave appliance cords hanging within reach of toddler.

- Avoid using microwave ovens to warm babies' milk. If you must use a microwave oven, always shake and test the temperature of the milk on the inside of your arm before feeding it to the baby.
- Keep hot dishes and hot drinks near the center of the table. Pass such dishes with care.
- Turn down your hot water heater to 120°F (49°C). Call your local utility company if you need help doing this.

Time For Skin to Burn at Different Temperatures	
Temperature	Burn Occurs Within
124°F (51°C)	4 minutes
131°F (55°C)	20 seconds
140°F (60°C)	5 seconds
150°F (65°C)	1 second

- Keep all cigarettes, matches, and lighters out of reach of children.
- Buy children's sleepwear, blankets, and bedding that is made of approved, fire-resistant fabric.
- Use protective screens around fireplaces and wood-burning stoves and make sure that the fire is out before going to bed or leaving the house.
- Install plastic covers over electrical outlets.
- Keep caustic and flammable chemicals out of reach of children. Lock them away.
- Use all the techniques to prevent fires that are discussed under Smoke Inhalation (see page *123*).
- Teach children how to drop and roll if their clothes become ignited with flames.
- Avoid sunburns by using sunscreen lotions and protective clothing.

BURNS

SYMPTOMS

- First-degree burn: reddened skin that is painful to the touch
- Second-degree burn: reddened or blotchy skin with blisters that is painful to the touch
- Third-degree burn: charred or white skin with deep tissue damage and injured nerve endings

TREATMENT

1. Monitor *A*irway, *B*reathing, and *C*irculation. Start CPR if necessary. (See page *24* for infants under one year of age; see page *41* for children aged one to eight.)

2. Treat the burns only after you establish that the child is breathing and has a pulse.

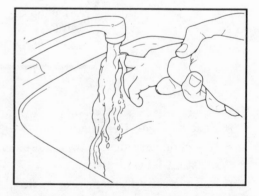

3. If small area is burned, immerse the area immediately in cool water.

4. If large area is burned, loosely apply clean, cool, damp dressings to the area.

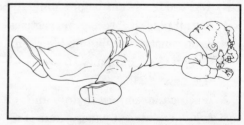

5. *Do not* place ice on the burn. Ice will cause more tissue damage. Cool water cools the tissue, but cold water or ice will cause the blood vessels to constrict, trapping the heat in the tissue and damaging it.

6. *Do not* use grease, oils, butter, or ointments on burns, as they retain heat and will cause more damage to the tissue.

7. *Do not* break blisters. You will be removing the protective layer of skin and increasing the risk of infection.

8. *Do not* remove the child's clothing if it is sticking to the burned skin.

9. *Do not* apply cotton.

10. *Do not* give the child anything to drink if he is unconscious. If he is conscious, consult with a physician.

11. For chemical burns, immediately put the child in a shower or bathtub or under a hose and flush the burned area with cool water. After the area is wet, remove the clothing, unless it is stuck to the skin.

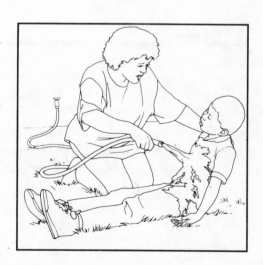

CHOKING

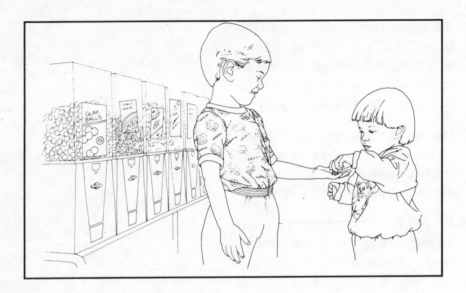

Choking is the most common cause of accidental death for children under one year of age and the most common cause of death in children under four years of age.

PREVENTION

- Mealtime should be a quiet time. Speaking while chewing should be discouraged. Running and walking while eating can increase the risk of inhalation of food and should be discouraged.
- Young children should not be given food that is the size or consistency of peanuts because the ability to chew and swallow is not well developed until about four years of age. Some examples of problem foods are nuts, raisins, peanut butter, hot dogs, grapes, apples, raw vegetables, and chunk-size pieces of meat. Young children should be given foods that dissolve or crumble in the mouth. Peanut butter should be spread thinly on bread or crackers; it should *never* be eaten from a spoon or finger.

- Children must be taught not to put objects other than food into their mouths.
- Examine the child's environment and remove all objects that are small enough for him to put into his mouth. Remove toys with detachable parts.
- Coins should not be given to young children as rewards or play items.
- Plastic bags and balloons can be easily inhaled or cause suffocation and should be disposed of appropriately.
- Crib bars should be no more than 2⅜ inches (6 centimeters) apart. (Federal safety regulations require that all cribs have this feature.) Broken side rails should be repaired immediately.
- Remove mobiles from the crib when the baby starts to grab for things, at approximately five months of age.
- Cribs should not have decorative poster extensions on their corners (required by Federal safety regulation). Children have tried to climb out of cribs, had clothing or string caught on the posters, and then strangled.
- Strings and cords should be kept out of the crib area.
- Cribs should not be placed near curtains or shades with cords.
- In other rooms remove all jewelry, ties, and sashes from the reach of children.
- Young babies should be placed on their sides or abdomen after feeding and should not be given a bottle in bed.

SYMPTOMS

- Child cannot cry or talk; no sound can be heard except for occasional high-pitched ineffective sounds
- Weak, ineffective cough
- Distressed breathing
- Inside of mouth may be blue
- Agitation
- Loss of consciousness (this is a severe, late sign of choking)

CHOKING

TREATMENT

1. **If the child is coughing effectively (you can hear the sound),** *do nothing* **except continue to observe.**

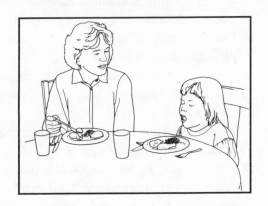

2. **If the cough is ineffective or respiratory distress worsens, monitor** *A*irway, *B*reathing, **and Circulation and perform the relief-of-choking skill for the conscious or unconscious infant or child. (See pages** *30–40* **or** *48–57*.)

3. *Do not* **place your fingers in the child's mouth to attempt to dislodge the object, as this may force the object farther down the airway. It also wastes time that could be used to perform the relief-of-choking skill.**

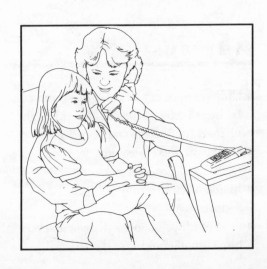

4. **Notify your physician after you perform the relief-of-choking skill, even if the child never lost consciousness and seems fine. Your physician may want to check that the object was not inhaled into the lung.**

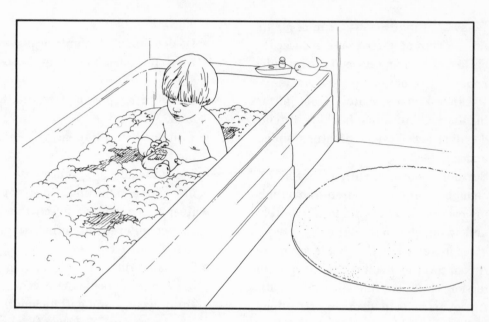

Drowning is the second most common cause of accidental death for children aged five to fourteen years in the United States. Most drownings occur in fresh water, and many children die within a few feet of safety. Approximately one-third of these drownings occur in the swimming pools of neighbors.

PREVENTION

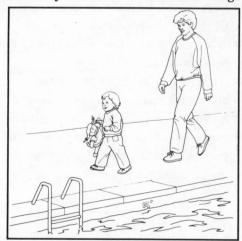

■ *Constant,* careful supervision of children near water is the *only* way to prevent drowning. Never leave a child alone in the water—not even for a few seconds. Take the child with you to answer the telephone, check the stove, answer the door, or use the bathroom.

DROWNING

- Be aware that drowning can occur in any amount of water that can cover the child's mouth and nose. This includes pools, lakes, oceans, ponds, rivers, streams, Jacuzzis, wading pools, gutters, birdbaths, fountains, buckets, ditches, dog dishes, fish tanks, bathtubs, sinks, and toilets.
- Surround your pool with a fence high enough to prevent children from climbing over it. Gates should latch securely and swing shut automatically. Keep gates locked when the pool is not in use. A pool cover by itself is not enough protection; children could slip underneath. A pool alarm is inadequate protection, as it could malfunction.
- Cover your pool or Jacuzzi with a hard cover when it is not in use.
- Keep a first-aid kit with instructions for CPR near the pool area.
- A telephone with list of emergency numbers should be near the pool.
- Have handy basic rescue devices (ring buoy with rope, rescue pole, large kickboard or other flat, floating board).
- Post a list of rules and make sure that your childen and their friends adhere to them. Some examples are:

- Never swim alone.
- Do not run, push, dunk, or play rough.
- Dive off the front of the diving board only.
- Do not bring glass objects into the pool area.
- Wait one hour after eating before entering the water.
- Leave the pool area immediately at the first sign of lightning or a storm.
- Keep toys and other objects that might attract children out of the pool and surrounding area.
- The same rules apply to wading pools as to swimming pools. Always watch the child. Empty and deflate small pools when not in use and turn them over so rain cannot collect in them.
- Never leave young children alone in the bathtub. If you must leave the bathroom take the child with you. Children can drown in a few inches of water if it covers their nose and mouth, and such an accident can happen quickly.
- Empty water buckets when not in use.
- Keep the lids of toilets down.
- Never leave water in a tub or basin.
- Turn off the filter system of a Jacuzzi when not in use.

■ Teach your child to swim. Knowing how
to swim will help him to feel relaxed,
confident, and competent in the water.
Remember that swimming or drown-
proofing skills are *never* a substitute for
constant supervision and *do not*, in
themselves, prevent drowning. Contact
your YMCA, YWCA, or community pool
for information about lessons.

SYMPTOMS

■ Obvious signs of distress in the water
■ Limp movements
■ Unconsciousness
■ Distressed breathing or no breathing at all
■ No pulse

TREATMENT

1. **Call out for help.**

2. **Try to reach the child from land or wade in and grab him. Do not let
him grab you. If you cannot reach the child directly, throw him
anything that will float (such as a buoy, kickboard, or log). If a**

rope is attached to the object,
throw the object beyond the child
and pull it into his reach.

3. If the child is too far away to
   reach, only an expert swimmer or
   certified lifeguard should swim
   toward the child with a float and
   grab him. If neither is available,
   call out for help and/or call 911.

4. Monitor *A*irway, *B*reathing, and
   *C*irculation. Start CPR if necessary. (See page *24* for infants
   under one year of age; see page *41*
   for children aged one to eight.)
   Rescue breathing may be performed while the child is still in
   the water.

5. If a child vomits, turn his head to
   the side. Clean out his mouth with
   your finger, reposition the airway,
   and continue CPR. If an infant
   under one year of age vomits, turn
   his whole body to the side, clean
   out his mouth, reposition the airway, and continue CPR. If you
   turn only the head of an infant
   you may block his airway.

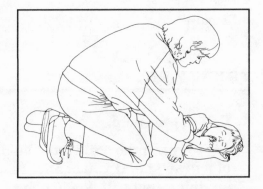

6. If a neck injury is suspected,
   CPR should be administered if
   necesary, but the jaw-lift maneu-

ver should be used to open the airway. If the jaw-lift maneuver does not work and you are unable to give breaths, tilt the head back to deliver breaths.

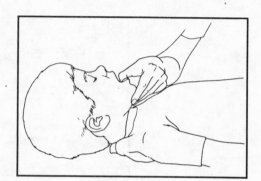

7. If the child falls through ice, calmly tell him (if conscious) not to try to climb out but to spread his arms over the top of the ice and to hold on. Reach the child by throwing any long object to him or by forming a human chain (each person lies spread-eagled on the ice and grabs the ankle of the person ahead of him). Have the child grab the object or hand and slide on his stomach to firm ice. Tell him not to walk. Grab the child if he is unconscious.

8. Once the child is revived, remove wet clothing and wrap him in blankets. If the child is hypothermic (extremely cold), he should be warmed slowly, under medical supervision.

9. Notify a physician any time breathing difficulty or a brief loss of consciousness occurs after a water accident, even if the child appears otherwise well.

ELECTRICAL SHOCK

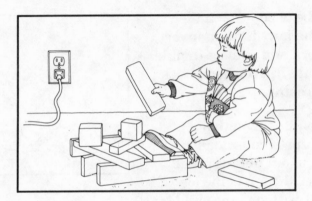

Electrical shock can cause a child to stop breathing. When you rescue a child who has sustained an electrical shock, you must protect yourself from also being shocked.

PREVENTION

- Be aware of your child's interest in electrical devices and cords.
- Cover electrical outlets. Covers can be purchased in most hardware stores or safety sections of variety stores, or outlets can be covered with electrical tape.
- Cover with electrical tape any cords lying on the floor that cannot be placed out of reach of children.
- Keep electrical appliances away from water.
- Unplug appliances when not in use.
- Teach children not to bite, chew, or play with electrical wires.

SYMPTOMS

- Child will be unconscious and may be in contact with the outlet, wire, or source of electricity.

TREATMENT

1. *DO NOT TOUCH THE CHILD DIRECTLY.* Be especially aware if the child is touching water or is near water because his body salt will make the water conduct the electricity, causing *you* to be shocked if you touch the child or the water.

2. Turn off electricity, if possible.

3. Break the child's contact with the electrical source without directly touching him. Use an object that will not carry an electrical charge, such as something made of rubber, wood, plastic, or paper. You could use a dry piece of wood, a board, a broom handle, a wooden spoon, a wooden baseball bat, a rubber shoe, a book, or a plastic ruler to knock the plug or wire or cord away from the child's body.

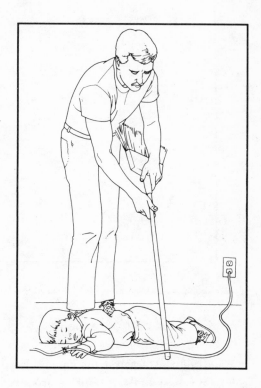

4. Monitor *A*irway, *B*reathing, and *C*irculation. Start CPR if necessary. (See page *24* for infants under one year of age; see page *41* for children aged one to eight.)

5. Treat for shock by elevating the legs, if possible, and covering the child with a blanket or clothes.

6. Treat for burns (see page *72*).

HEAD, NECK, AND BACK INJURIES

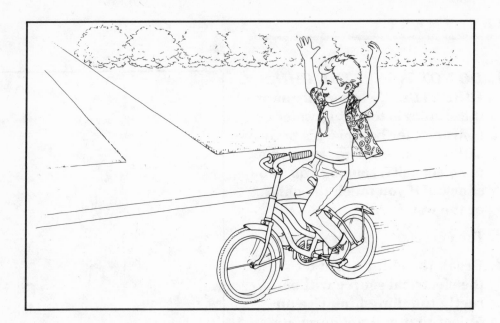

Head injuries account for nearly 250,000 hospital admissions each year. The most common causes of head injuries are automobile accidents, bicycle accidents, and falls from furniture, stairs, and while at play. Most neck and back (spinal cord) injuries result from being struck by an object, thrown by force, or falling. If a child has a head injury, a neck or back injury should also be suspected.

PREVENTION

- Always use car seats or restraints in the car.
- Supervise your child at play, especially when he is playing on swings, slides, or is swimming.

- Set limits with children about where, when, and how to dive safely into a pool or body of water.
- Use net gates at stairs if you have a baby or toddler.
- Keep stairs safe by clearing them of toys, laundry, and other items. Keep them repaired. Remove or repair loose carpeting or treads, and install secure handrails at child and adult levels. Do not use the stairs as a storage area.
- Do not allow a toddler to play in a walker near stairs.
- Encourage a child to wear a helmet while riding a bicycle. Teach your child bicycle safety, including where to ride, how fast, and how to obey traffic rules (see Injuries: Miscellaneous, page *108*).
- Install nonskid surfaces in bathtubs and showers.
- Teach children not to jump or play on furniture.
- Anchor all rugs.
- Keep siderails of a crib up and consider moving the child to a bed when he has the ability to stand and climb on siderails.
- Provide good lighting in your environment.
- Install safety glass or plastic on sliding glass doors and on windows near doors or stairs. Mark glass doors with decals.
- Install locks that limit window opening. Do not allow children to play on windowsills.
- Clean spills immediately and do not overwax floors.
- Do not leave a baby unattended on a changing table or bed.
- Use an infant seat properly and do not leave a baby alone in it.
- Purchase a sturdy high chair with a safety belt attached to the frame. Use the safety belt whenever the child is in the chair.
- Keep the electric garage door switch out of reach of children. Purchase a door that reverses when any resistance is met, and keep it well lubricated.
- Use only toy boxes with slow-closing, hinged lids. Ask someone at your local hardware store for these hinges.
- Make sure that all toys are put away after playtime, both indoors and out.
- Remove or pad all furniture with sharp edges or glass tops.

HEAD, NECK, AND BACK INJURIES

SYMPTOMS OF NECK OR BACK INJURY

- Pain in neck or back
- Possible paralysis
- Body in an odd or deformed position
- Cuts and bruises
- Swelling (in later stages)
- Signs of head injury

SYMPTOMS OF A HEAD INJURY

- Change in behavior: dizziness, weakness, numbness, difficulty breathing, convulsions, unconsciousness
- Vomiting and headache
- Deformity of the skull
- Open scalp wound
- Loss of bowel or bladder control
- Blood or clear fluid running from the ears, nose, or mouth
- Pupils of unequal size
- Fever above 101°F (38°C)

TREATMENT

1. Monitor *Airway*, *Breathing*, and *Circulation*. Start CPR if necessary. (See page *24* for infants under one year of age; see page *41* for children aged one to eight.) Use the jaw-lift maneuver if you need to open the airway to give breaths.

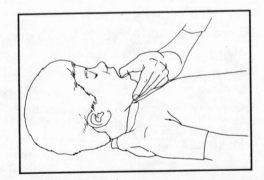

2. Do not move the child unless it is absolutely necessary; that is, if the area is dangerous or you must start CPR. If you must move or turn the child, turn him as a straight unit, as though he were a log, keeping his head in line with his spinal column. Keep the child from moving if he is conscious. If a child has a head injury, a neck or back injury should also be suspected.

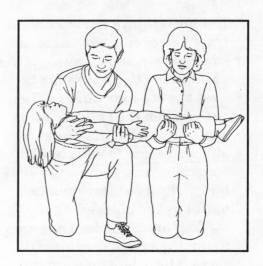

3. Immobilize the head, neck, and back to prevent any movement by using blankets or pillows on the sides of the child.

4. Keep the child warm and quiet.

5. Treat bleeding if necessary (see page *66*).

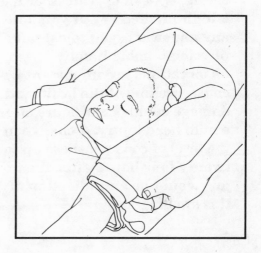

6. If possible, record the child's symptoms, level of consciousness, and time that you discovered the injury.

7. If a head injury causes only a brief loss of consciousness, notify a physician and awaken the child every two hours for the first twenty-four hours. When you awaken the child, ask him some questions that he can usually answer, to test his level of consciousness. If the child is a baby, observe him when he awakens for his feeding or awaken him if he does not wake up on time for a feeding. Observe if he is less interested in eating, is weak or listless, or has a high-pitched cry. If you note any abnormal symptoms, call a physician immediately. These observations are important because swelling of the brain and damage could occur hours after a mild head injury. A change in the level of consciousness up to twenty-four hours after the injury could be an indication of this swelling.

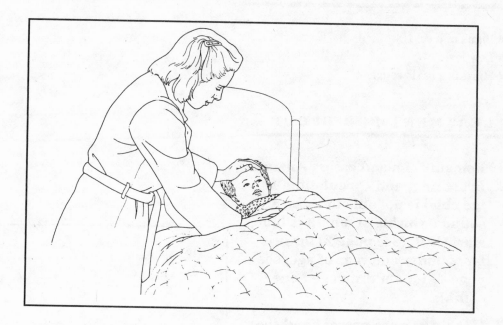

Although the majority of upper-airway infections do not result in a complete airway obstruction, such blockage can occur during the course of certain infections. The most common infections that can result in airway obstructions are croup and epiglottitis.

CROUP

Croup, an infection of the trachea and back of the throat, occurs more frequently than epiglottitis, and is usually less serious. It is caused by a virus and occurs in children from about six months to three years of age. Its symptoms arise slowly, and a child usually will not be very ill.

INFECTIONS OF THE UPPER AIRWAY (CROUP AND EPIGLOTTITIS)

SYMPTOMS OF CROUP

- Signs of a cold
- Low fever
- "Barking seal" cough

TREATMENT FOR CROUP

1. **Remain calm and assess *A*irway, *B*reathing, and *C*irculation. If the child is not able to make a sound or inside of mouth is blue, start CPR. (See page *24* for infants under one year of age; see page *41* for children aged one to eight.)**

2. **If the *ABC*s are present and the child is still able to make sounds, provide humidity. You can do this by turning on a hot shower and having the child sit in the bathroom with the door closed, by giving cool mist if you have a humidifier, or by taking the child outside if there is fog or rain.**

3. **Call a physician if the child's airway is partially obstructed and he *can* still make sounds or speak.**

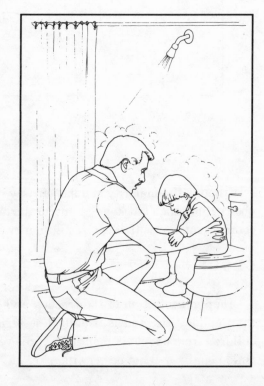

EPIGLOTTITIS

Epiglottitis is a serious, life-threatening condition. It is an infection of the epiglottis, the flap of tissue that covers the windpipe when you swallow. It is caused by bacteria and usually occurs in children who are older than two years of age. Its symptoms arise quickly, and a child will usually become very ill. If the epiglottis becomes swollen, it can cause a *complete* airway obstruction.

SYMPTOMS OF EPIGLOTTITIS

- High fever
- Sore throat
- Drooling
- Child leans forward and sticks out his chin to open the airway and to relieve the pain of swallowing

TREATMENT OF EPIGLOTTITIS

1. Monitor *A*irway, *B*reathing, and *C*irculation. If the child cannot make a sound, start CPR. (See page *24* for infants under one year of age; see page *41* for children aged one to eight.) Try to give breaths even if you think

INFECTIONS OF THE UPPER AIRWAY (CROUP AND EPIGLOTTITIS)

the airway is totally obstructed. If the child becomes unconscious, you will have a better chance of delivering breaths because the muscles of the throat will relax.

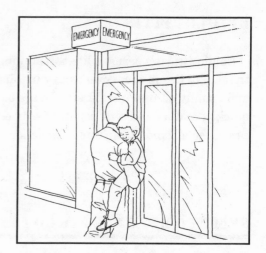

2. Remain calm. If you are anxious and cause the child to cry, the epiglottis could swell, causing a complete airway obstruction.

3. If the child can make a sound and a partial obstruction is present, bring the child to the emergency room. Call 911 if the obstruction is complete and the child cannot make a sound.

4. Do not put anything into the child's throat, as this may cause a partial obstruction to become a complete obstruction.

5. Do not perform the relief-of-choking skill unless you think that there is an object in the airway.

INFECTIOUS DISEASE IN DAY-CARE CENTERS AND SCHOOLS

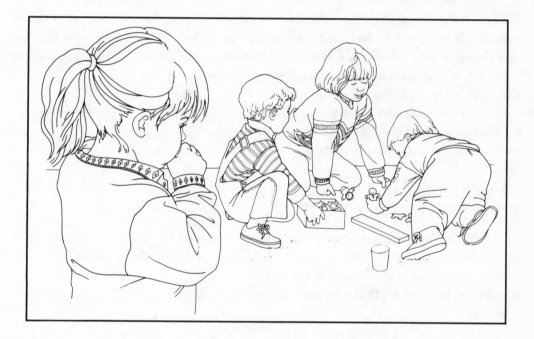

It is estimated that eleven million children in the United States receive part-time or full-time care by individuals other than their parents. The majority of this care is given in day-care centers.

Young children in day-care centers and older children in school are at risk for infection because of their immature defenses against disease and their increased exposure to infection. It may be possible to reduce a child's risk of acquiring infection and disease by knowing about risk factors, transmission, common diseases, and proper preventive practices.

INFECTIOUS DISEASE IN DAY-CARE CENTERS AND SCHOOLS

RISK FACTORS

The amount of infection in a day-care center or school is related to the degree that the infection is present in the community. Children at greatest risk for infection are infants and toddlers who have had limited exposure to infection prior to attending day care and who are still wearing diapers. Specific characteristics of day-care centers or schools that lead to an increased risk of infection are:

- The presence of children in diapers
- Close, repeated person-to-person contact among the children
- Frequent exploration of environment with mouths
- Hands-on contact of staff members and teachers.

TRANSMISSION

Whether or not a disease is spread depends on how bad the germ is, on hygiene, on how many children are cared for together, and on how young the children are. A disease can be spread in the following ways:

- From the feces (stool) to the mouth via hands
- In food
- From direct, person-to-person contact
- Through the air
- From contact with toys, utensils, or surfaces contaminated with the infectious organism
- Prenatally, when the fetus becomes infected from an infected pregnant woman.

PRACTICES TO PREVENT INFECTION

1. Hand washing is the *best* way to prevent the spread of disease. All staff members should wash their hands:

- After arrival at the center or school
- After changing diapers
- After helping a child use the toilet
- After using the toilet themselves
- After wiping or blowing noses
- Before preparing food.

Hands should be washed with a pump-type soap dispenser and dried with paper towels. The water faucet should be turned off with a paper towel (not with clean hands).

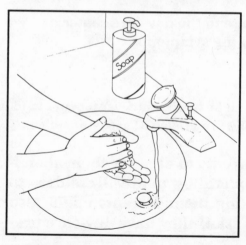 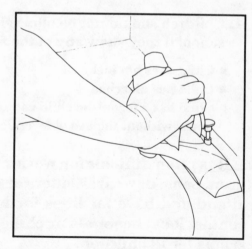

2. Properly dispose of soiled articles.

- Place diapers in plastic bags in a plastic-lined garbage pail.
- Place dirty or soiled clothes or linen in plastic bags.
- Laundering should not be done at the center or school, to avoid accumulation of soiled linen.

3. **All items used by or around children should be properly and regularly cleaned.**

   - Potty chairs should not be rinsed in sinks. They should be rinsed in the toilet.
   - Wash a changing table with disinfectant, such as a solution of diluted bleach that is one part bleach, nine parts water, using paper towels, after each use.
   - Ideally, the staff members who change diapers should not prepare food.
   - If nonpaper dishware is used, it should be washed in a dishwasher, located in the kitchen.
   - Soiled clothes should not be rinsed in the kitchen.
   - Toys should be cleaned every day with a disinfectant, such as a solution of diluted bleach that is one part bleach, nine parts water.
   - Uncarpeted floors should be disinfected regularly.

4. **Children should not be allowed to attend the day-care center or school if they show any of the following symptoms:**

   - Child does not feel well.
   - Child has diarrhea.
   - Child has a fever (the child can return if he is without fever for twenty-four hours without the use of fever-reducing drugs such as acetominophen).

It is often difficult for working parents to care for their ill children. Some day-care centers or schools allow mildly ill children to attend and have facilities for isolating them. Parents might also contact local hospitals or clinics to ask if they have day-care programs for ill children.

5. **Children should not be allowed to attend the day-care center or school unless they have received the required vaccinations. The following is an immunization schedule for children beginning immunization in early infancy.**

AGE	VACCINES
2 months (6–10 weeks)	DTP and OPV (OPV may be started at this age even for premature and/or low-birthweight infants who are otherwise well.)
4 months	DTP and OPV
6 months	DTP (An additional OPV dose at this time is optional in areas of high risk for polio exposure.)
15 months	MMR
15–18 months	DTP and OPV (If child has not received MMR, it can be given simultaneously with DTP and OPV, at separate sites.)
18 months	Hib (Hib may be given to some high-risk children as early as age 18 months or as late as five years.)
4–6 years (before school entry)	DTP and OPV
14–16 years (and every 10 years thereafter)	Td

KEY

DTP:	Diphtheria, Tetanus, Pertussis	MMR:	Measles, Mumps, and Rubella
OPV:	Oral Polio Vaccine	Hib:	Hemophilus Influenzae
		Td:	Tetanus

INFECTIOUS DISEASE IN DAY-CARE CENTERS AND SCHOOLS

COMMON CHILDHOOD DISEASES

The charts on the following pages outline the most common diseases a child may get. Included are the symptoms of the disease, how the disease is acquired, and possible ways to treat it and/or prevent its spread.

RESPIRATORY OR FLULIKE DISEASES

Disease	Organism	Symptoms	Transmission	Prevention/ Treatment	Comment
Respiratory viral infections	Respiratory syncytial virus Parainfluenza virus Influenza virus Adenovirus Rhinovirus Enterovirus	Runny nose, cough, sore throat, occasional fever	Respiratory droplets, direct contact	Rest, supportive care	Most young children have 2–8 upper-respiratory infections each year. Usually children do not become very ill. If outbreak is prolonged, it is important to check sick people to be sure that illness is not caused by bacteria that can be treated with antibiotics. Be aware that such illness may cause ear infection.
Hemophilus influenza type B	*Hemophilus influenzae* type B bacteria	Runny nose, cough, sore throat, nausea, vomiting, diarrhea, fever	Respiratory droplets, direct contact; most cases occur in children under age 5.	Vaccine available for children older than 18 months. Spread may be prevented by treatment with the drug rifampin.	If disease is identified, all parents should be notified.

RESPIRATORY OR FLULIKE DISEASES (continued)

Disease	Organism	Symptoms	Transmission	Prevention/Treatment	Comment
Meningococcal meningitis	*Neisseria meningitidis* bacteria	Fever, nausea, vomiting, headache	Respiratory droplets, direct contact; children under 1 year of age are at increased risk.	Vaccine is available but does not protect against all types of the bacteria. Vaccine is for children older than 2 years of age. Rifampin may protect against spread of disease.	If disease is identified, notify public health department officials.
Group A streptococcus	Group A *streptococcus* bacteria	Fever, runny nose, sore throat	Direct contact	Antibiotics	Infected children should be excluded from day-care center or school until treated with antibiotics for 24 hours.
Tuberculosis	*Mycobacterium tuberculosis*	Fever, malaise, cough	Respiratory droplets; infected children are usually not more contagious than infected adults.	Antituberculosis drugs	If disease is identified, contact public health department officials. Adult workers should be screened for tuberculosis before starting work. Children should be excluded from day-care center or school until drug therapy is started.

DIARRHEAL DISEASES

Disease	Organism	Symptoms	Transmission	Prevention/Treatment	Comment
Hepatitis A	Hepatitis A virus	Diarrhea, fever, malaise, jaundice	Stool-mouth, water, direct contact, possibly surfaces. Common in day-care centers with children under 2 years. Children do not but adults can become very ill. Can be contagious without symptoms.	Immunoglobulin to prevent further spread.	Immunoglobulin may interfere with some vaccines such as the Measles-Mumps-Rubella (MMR) vaccine.
Shigellosis	Shigella bacteria	Diarrhea	Direct contact, food, water. Usually affects children aged 1 to 5. People with symptoms are more likely to transmit the disease.	Antibiotics may improve symptoms and decrease the chance of carrying the disease. Antidiarrheal agents may only prolong the course of the disease.	If this disease is identified, stool cultures from others in contact with the sick person should be checked. Infected persons should be kept out of the day-care center or school until 3 cultures of stool samples show no growth of shigellae.

DIARRHEAL DISEASES (continued)

Disease	Organism	Symptoms	Transmission	Prevention/Treatment	Comment
Salmonellosis	*Salmonella* bacteria	Diarrhea	Direct contact, food. Babies under 1 year of age are at greatest risk but persons of all ages may be affected. Small children may not have symptoms but can transmit the disease.	Antibiotics are not usually recommended because they may promote resistant strains of the bacteria.	Stool cultures from others in contact with the sick person should be checked. Infected persons should be kept out of school until 3 cultures of stool samples show no growth of salmonellae.
Campylobacter enteritis	*Campylobacter jejuni* bacteria	Diarrhea	Direct contact, food, possibly stool-mouth. People may carry the germ without having symptoms.	Erythromycin may decrease the time that a person will carry the disease.	Children who have symptoms should be kept out of the day-care center or school.
Giardiasis	*Giardia lamblia* protozoan parasite	Diarrhea	Stool-mouth, water, and surfaces contaminated by stool. Infection without symptoms is common.	Treat with anti-Giardia drugs such as quinacrin hydrochloride, metronidazole, or furazolidone.	Stool specimens of all people in contact with infected persons should be cultured. People with symptoms should be excluded from the day-care center or school. Isolation of infected people without symptoms is controversial.

DISEASES PREVENTABLE BY VACCINATION

Disease	Organism	Symptoms	Transmission	Prevention/Treatment	Comment
Measles	Rubeola virus	Fever, weakness, rash	Respiratory droplets and secretions, direct contact, possibly surfaces. Most contagious before rash. Children in day-care centers are at highest risk for the disease.	MMR vaccine	Children with measles should be sent home for 5 days after rash appears. Staff and children without vaccination should be excluded until they receive vaccine or immunoglobulin. Vaccine is good within 72 hours of exposure. Immunoglobulin is good within 6 days of exposure.
Mumps	Mumps virus	Fever, swollen neck glands	Respiratory droplets, direct contact. Contagious 1 week before to 9 days after swelling of neck glands.	MMR vaccine	Exclude from day-care center or school until swelling is gone. Vaccine is for children older than 12 months.

DISEASES PREVENTABLE BY VACCINATION

Disease	Organism	Symptoms	Transmission	Prevention/ Treatment	Comment
Rubella (German measles)	Rubella virus	Fever, weakness, rash	Respiratory droplets, direct contact, surfaces. Children in day-care centers are at highest risk for contracting disease.	MMR vaccine	Infected persons should be excluded for 5 days after rash appears. Men and women of child-bearing years as well as children should be vaccinated. Any identified cases should be reported to public health department officials. Pregnant women should not be vaccinated. Pregnant women exposed to virus may want their blood tested for presence of the virus.
Pertussis (whooping cough)	*Bordetella pertussis* bacteria	Fever, weakness, cough	Respiratory droplets, direct contact. Contagious when coughing begins and until 4 weeks after cough is gone.	Vaccine. Antibiotics may decrease time that person is contagious. Antibiotics may protect others from becoming infected.	

OTHER VIRUSES

Disease	Organism	Symptoms	Transmission	Prevention/Treatment	Comment
Chicken pox (varicella)	Varicella-zoster virus	Fever, weakness, rash	Respiratory droplets. Child is contagious 2 days before and 6 days after rash. Eleven- to 20-day incubation period.		Infected children should stay home for 1 week after first lesion appears.
Cytomegalovirus infection	Cytomegalovirus	Weakness, sore throat, runny nose, occasional fever	Secretions, excretions (urine and stool), direct contact, possibly surfaces. Usually carriers do not have symptoms. Children 12–24 months are most likely to become infected.	Proper handwashing	The risk is that infection will spread to pregnant women and the unborn baby to cause birth defects.
AIDS (acquired immune deficiency syndrome)	HIV	Signs of weakened immune defenses.	Sexual contact, sharing contaminated needles, through placental blood to fetus of infected pregnant women, through infected blood supplies. No evidence at this time that virus can be transmitted through casual contact.	For those who are sexually active and for those who use needles: Use of condoms during sexual intercourse. No sharing of needles. Clean needles with bleach solution.	The AIDS virus cannot be contracted through casual contact. If concern remains about surface contact, a bleach solution is an effective, inexpensive substance to use as a disinfectant and kills the AIDS virus instantly.

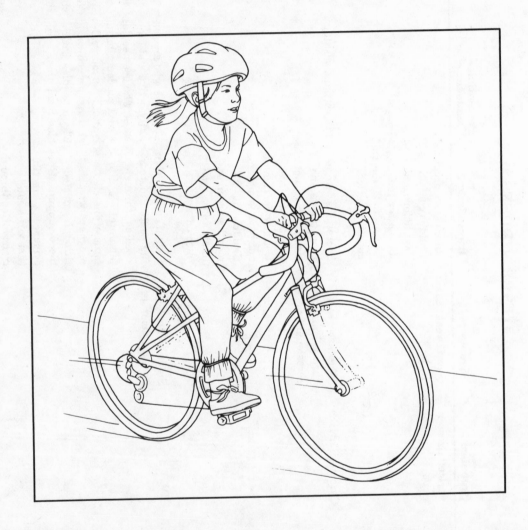

Injuries, the leading cause of death during childhood, occur both in and out of the home. In this book the most common injuries are discussed separately. Other causes of injury to children occur less frequently but are serious enough to deserve mention. Preventive measures for these injuries will be suggested. Treatment for a few less common, but serious, problems will be described.

ANIMALS

- Do not assume that your dog will not bite. It may be jealous of the baby or may not be used to children's rough play. Never leave the dog and child alone. Make sure that your dog's shots are up to date. Dog bites can cause infections that can be fatal. The majority of dog bites each year are caused by dogs owned by the victim's family. One-third of the victims are babies less than one year of age, bitten in a crib.
- Teach children not to approach nervous, strange, or injured animals, even their own. They should not touch any animal that they do not know.
- Teach children to treat all animals with kindness and respect. Any animal can bite or scratch if mistreated or frightened.

BATTERIES

- The small disc-shaped batteries used for cameras, calculators, watches, and the like may cause blockage of the airway if inhaled. The leaking chemicals may cause burns of the airway, stomach, and blood vessels, resulting in tissue damage and bleeding. Discard old batteries so that children cannot find them, and keep new batteries out of the reach of children.

BICYCLES

- Make sure that your child's bicycle is the right size and style for his age, height, and skill. Employees at your local bike shop should be able to help you make the right selection. Be sure your child accompanies you when it is time to fit the height of the seat and the angle of the handlebars.
- Make sure the bicycle is in good working order. Employees at your local bike shop should be able to help you.

■ Once the child has learned the basics of balance and riding a bicycle, enroll him in a bicycle safety and training program. Such programs are usually sponsored by your local police, YMCA/YWCA, automobile association, or community recreation department, and they emphasize skill as well as road safety. If no such program is available, you must make sure that your child understands all traffic rules and regulations. A bicycle is a vehicle, and the rider is required by law to observe certain rules and regulations. These rules are available at your local Department of Motor Vehicles. The following are some basic rules for bicycle riders:

1. Always wear an approved safety helmet.
2. Use a light and wear white or reflective clothing at night.
3. Use a clip or other tie device on pant cuffs.
4. Keep to the right and ride with traffic, not against it.
5. Signal all stops and turns with the proper arm signals.
6. Ride single file.
7. Watch for car doors opening and for cars pulling out into traffic.
8. Walk bikes across intersections.
9. Stop for all red lights and stop signs, as a car would.
10. Keep both hands on the handlebars.
11. Do not carry other riders on the handlebars, cross bars, seat, or fenders.
12. Be especially alert for others on hills and curves.

■ Set limits on where the child can ride. Even older children can become overtired or lost if they ride too far from home. They should always let you know if they are traveling beyond a few blocks from home.

CAMPING

■ Outdoor hikes and camping trips should always have adult supervision. Make sure that the trip is not beyond the child's level of skill or endurance, and plan for adequate food, water, shelter, and clothing. Bring a compass, working flashlight, and whistle. Expect the unexpected and be prepared for rain, insects, sudden cold, or severe sun. Always take a first-aid kit, including treatment for insect bites. More information about camping and survival skills can be found in books about those subjects and is taught in special scouting, camping, and hiking programs.

GLASS

- Install safety glass or plastic windows and doors whenever possible and make glass doors more visible with decals.
- Keep drinking glasses and other glass objects away from young childen. Use plastic cups and plates.
- Keep glass decorations and Christmas tree ornaments out of reach of young children.

GUNS

- Most accidental deaths of children in the home are caused by misuse of real guns. The group most frequently involved is boys less than five years of age. Children are interested in guns because their heroes on television, in the movies, and in cartoons use them. If you must own a gun, always keep it locked and out of the sight and reach of children. Lock the bullets in a separate location. Do not buy toy guns for a child.

PLAYGROUND

- Do not allow the child to play in playgrounds where the equipment is not safe or is beyond his level of strength and skill. Make sure that your child understands which equipment he can and cannot use. Do not allow the child to play where there is broken glass, aluminum pull tabs, rubbish, old lumber and nails, animal feces, or other debris.

PLAYPEN

- If you use a playpen, make sure that the slats are close enough together to prevent the child's head from being caught in between. They should be less than 2⅜ inches (6 centimeters) apart. Mesh nets should be tear-proof, with holes closely spaced. Playpens are not meant to serve as babysitters. You still must supervise the child while he is in the playpen.

STRANGERS

- Accompany the child on frequently traveled routes (to and from school and friends' houses) to make sure that he knows the accepted route and its particular hazards. Work with neighbors to appoint one or two "safe homes," and explain to the child what to do if an accident or emergency happens.
- Teach your child not to accept rides, gifts, or candy from a stranger, and not to go anywhere with a stranger.

TOYS

- Never give coins as rewards or play items.
- Before buying any toy, examine it with your child's safety in mind. Always look for simplicity of design and quality of material and construction. Buy toys that will withstand repetitive use, and check toys regularly to make sure that rough edges and other interior construction devices have not become exposed.
- Allow the child to play only with toys appropriate for his age and ability. Do not allow a child to play with an older sibling's toys.
- Do not purchase toys with removable or sharp parts, with cords longer than twelve inches (thirty centimeters), or with dangerous hinges or metal edges.
- Teach children not to run with sharp objects in their hands nor with any objects in their mouths.

TRAFFIC

■ Teach children proper traffic safety:

1. Never hitchhike or accept rides with strangers.
2. Walk on the sidewalk.
3. If it is necessary to walk in the street, walk on the side facing oncoming traffic and be particularly alert on hills and around curves.
4. Look both ways before crossing the street, and cross only at corners or crosswalks.
5. Obey traffic signals and signs, and listen to policemen, student patrol guards, and crossing guards.

POISONING

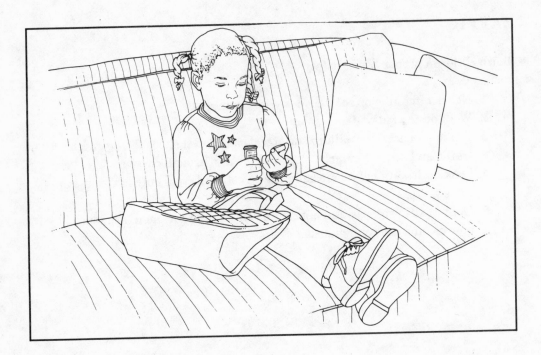

Poisoning is the fourth most common cause of death of young children. One million cases are reported each year, with 3,000 deaths. Poisoning occurs most frequently in children one to four years of age. There are three ways in which poisoning can occur: ingestion (swallowing), inhalation (breathing), and contact (touching).

PREVENTION

- Keep all medications, poisons, perfumes, cosmetics, and other chemicals out of the reach of children and away from food. Do not put them on the bedside stand, kitchen table, or bathroom counter for convenience. Lock them up if possible.

- Throw away all old medicines by flushing them down the toilet.
- Label all medications appropriately and leave them in their original containers. Read all labels and follow instructions carefully.
- Avoid taking medicine in the presence of children, as they like to imitate adults.
- Keep all medication out of purses and keep purses out of reach of children. Be conscious of other people's purses when you visit someone else's home or when visitors come to your home. Children find purses fascinating and are readily attracted to them.
- Do not assume that childproof containers cannot be opened by children.
- Always turn on the light when measuring or pouring medicine.
- Never call medicine "candy."
- Warn children not to eat or drink medications, chemicals, plants, or berries that they may find. Teach your child at an early age that some of these pretty items are dangerous.
- Keep toxic household plants out of the house and yard. Check the toxic plant list on page *135* to see which plants are poisonous, and consult with experts at the poison control center or at your local nursery. When in doubt, get them out!
- Wash hands and cover cuts when preparing food and cooking. Your hands may have germs on them that can cause food poisoning.
- Do not eat or serve foods that smell bad or look spoiled. Young children may have immature stomachs and lack immunity to germs. Even leftovers that may be fine for adults might make a young child ill.
- Do not feed babies raw honey; it contains spores that may cause botulism poisoning in a young child.
- Store food properly to prevent *Staphylococcus aureus* infections. Keep hot food hot and cold food cold. Defrost frozen foods in the refrigerator, not on the counter. Do not leave food that could spoil at room temperature.
- Cook foods properly, especially meats, eggs, milk, and poultry, to prevent salmonella poisoning.
- Cool leftover soups, stews, and meats in refrigerator, *not* at room temperature, before storing. Boil gravy before serving to prevent *Clostridium perfringens* poisoning.

POISONING

- Do not store poisonous substances in food or beverage containers; for example, never store paint thinner in a soft drink bottle. Children associate these containers with food.
- Use cleaning fluids in an area with good ventilation.
- Do not build with asbestos, and check old homes for asbestos insulation.
- Do not allow children to play in or with any type of insulation.
- Check furniture, carpet, and clothing labels for presence of formaldehyde; do not purchase items that contain it.
- To prevent lead poisoning, discourage toddlers from eating dirt or paint chips.
- Have your furnace and hot-water heater checked yearly to prevent carbon monoxide poisoning.
- Do not leave children in a car with the engine running.
- **Have on hand two bottles per child of syrup of ipecac, which is used to induce vomiting when appropriate.** It can be purchased at any drugstore. (We recommend that you buy two bottles per child if your children are older than one year because they might need more than one dose, and because sometimes more than one child will swallow poisonous substances.)
- **Some authorities recommend having activated charcoal on hand in the home.** The use of this substance remains controversial. It is known to be effective in absorbing some poisonous substances, but it is difficult to give to children because of its form and bad flavor. Discuss the use of it with your pediatrician before purchasing it.

SYMPTOMS

Ingested Poisons

- Information from witnesses or child
- Empty containers or bottles
- Burns around the mouth or on the hands
- Nausea, stomach pain, or cramps
- Drowsiness or loss of consciousness

- Difficulty breathing—shallow, heavy, or labored breaths
- Seizures
- With petroleum poisoning: burning, coughing, gagging, coma, petrol odor on breath

Inhaled Poisons

- Situation in which the child is found
- Information from witnesses
- Irritation of eyes, throat, or lungs
- Coughing
- Headache
- Nausea and vomiting
- Dizziness
- Breathing difficulty or absence of breathing
- Confusion, difficulty awakening, or unconsciousness
- With carbon monoxide poisoning: cherry red, then blue color

Contact Poisons

- Burning and itching
- Rash
- Swelling
- Blisters
- Headache
- Fever
- Some poisons (such as rat poison) are absorbed through the skin so burns may not be seen.

TREATMENT

Ingested Poisons

1. **Watch the child's *Airway*, *Breathing*, and *Circulation*. Start CPR if necessary. (See page *24* for infants under one year of age;**

see page *41* for children aged one to eight.)

2. **Call the poison control center. Be prepared to tell them:**

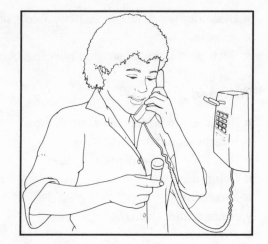

   - Age and weight of the child
   - What was ingested—take the container to the telephone with you
   - When it was ingested
   - How much was ingested
   - How the child is feeling or acting right now
   - Your name and telephone number.

3. **If instructed to do so by the experts at the poison control center, give the child a glass of water or milk.**

4. **If directed to induce vomiting, use syrup of ipecac:**

   - Small child: give ½ ounce (15 milliliters) with 8 ounces (250 milliliters) of water, as marked on the bottle.
   - Large child: give 1 ounce (30 milliliters) with 8 ounces (250 mililiters) of water as marked on the bottle.
   - Repeat after twenty minutes if vomiting has not occurred and you are advised to repeat the dose.

5. ***Never* induce vomiting unless instructed to do so by experts at the poison control center. *Never* induce vomiting unless the child is conscious. Some substances can burn the tissue inside the throat and lungs when vomited. *Do not* induce vomiting if:**

   - The child is unconscious
   - You see burns around the mouth or on the hands
   - You smell gasoline
   - The child is having seizures or is exhausted.

6. *Do not* follow the antidotes on labels of poisonous substances, as they can be outdated or inaccurate. Call the poison control center.

Inhaled Poisons

1. Move the child into fresh air. Open doors and windows. Avoid inhaling the fumes yourself.

2. Call the poison control center.

3. Monitor *Airway,* *Breathing,* and *Circulation.* Start CPR and call 911 if necessary. (See page *24* for infants under age one; see page *41* for children aged one to eight.)

Contact Poisons

1. Do not remove clothing if it sticks to the skin or is difficult to remove. Wash the area with a large amount of water. You can use a shower, bath, hose, or sink to do this.

2. If poison is in the eye, flush the eye with large amounts of cool water.

3. Call the poison control center to ask for further advice.

POISON TREATMENT SUMMARY

1. Identify the type of poison

2. Call poison control center

3. Dilute

4. Observe the child

5. Call your physician

SEIZURES CAUSED BY FEVER

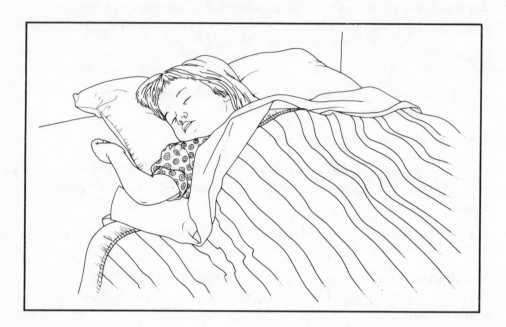

Seizures caused by fever (febrile seizures) are relatively common among children aged six months to five years. Approximately 3 to 4 percent of all children younger than five years of age have febrile seizures. They generally are not life threatening and do not mean that the child has epilepsy. Some children have one febrile seizure and never have another, whereas other young children react to every fever with a seizure.

Febrile seizures occur because a sudden rise in temperature sets off an erratic electrical activity in the brain. All the brain cells send messages independently to the muscles of the body, and the muscles contract violently. This is what you see as the fit or convulsion. It is important to remember that it is the sudden rise of the temperature, not how high it is, that causes the seizure to occur.

SYMPTOMS

Phase 1 (tonic phase): this usually lasts about ten to twenty seconds.

- Loud, high-pitched cry
- Extension of the arms and legs
- Rigid body
- Eyes rolled back
- Frothing at the mouth
- Falling to the ground
- Loss of consciousness

Phase 2 (clonic phase): this usually lasts about thirty seconds. It is also called a fit or convulsion.

- Jerking movements

Phase 3 (deep sleep): this usually lasts minutes to hours. All of the muscles have just worked very hard and the child is tired.

- Periods of deep sleep

TREATMENT

1. Monitor *Airway*, *Breathing*, and *Circulation*. Start CPR if the child stops breathing after the seizure has stopped. (See page *24* for infants under one year of age; see page *41* for children aged one to eight.)

2. Do not restrain the child.

3. Move furniture out of the way so the child will not be injured.

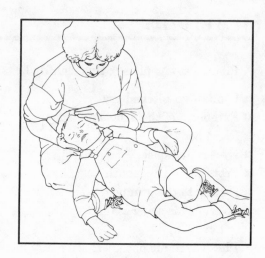

4. Maintain the airway during the seizure but turn the head or body (if an infant) to the side if vomiting occurs.

5. *Do not* put anything into the mouth. You may injure the child's mouth, or the child may bite you. A person cannot swallow a tongue. The airway will not become blocked if the head is positioned properly, with the ears and nose in an imaginary line perpendicular to the floor.

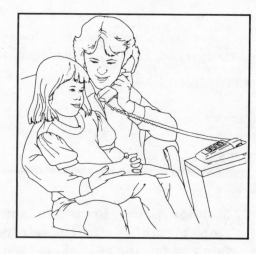

6. Notify a physician after the seizure is over and the child is breathing.

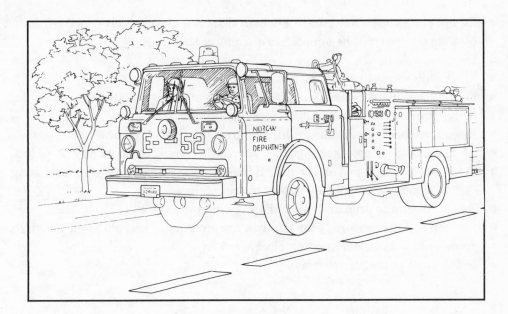

Smoke inhalation accounts for four out of five deaths related to fires. It is most often deadly when toxic fumes are created by the burning of synthetic materials, such as nylon, vinyl, and polyurethane.

PREVENTION

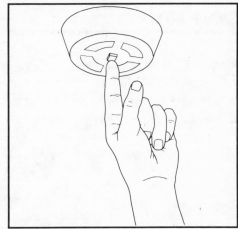

- Never leave small children home alone.
- Purchase and install smoke detectors in the hall outside of the bedrooms. Regularly check them to make sure that they work by using the check button provided, or use Safe Smoke spray (recommended in *Consumer Reports*).

SMOKE INHALATION

- Do not place smoke detector in kitchen, since it will sound with smoke from cooking and you will be tempted to disconnect it.
- Do not smoke in bed.
- Teach children not to play with matches.
- Do not leave matches or lighters within reach of young children.
- Never store flammable liquids in glass containers.
- Regularly check your home for hidden fire hazards and remove them.
- Close doors to bedrooms at night to prevent the spread of smoke in case of fire.
- Teach children to crawl on the floor if there is heavy smoke, to avoid breathing carbon monoxide, and to close doors in event of fire.
- Teach children to drop and roll if their clothing is on fire.
- Develop and discuss with your family a fire emergency exit plan and identify a predetermined outdoor meeting place.
- In the event of fire, remember:

> *F*ind
> *I*nform
> *R*estrict
> *E*xit

SYMPTOMS

- Visible fire or smoke
- Soot on face or clothes
- Difficulty breathing
- Burns

TREATMENT

1. Remove the child and yourself from immediate danger and into fresh air.

2. Call out for help. Shout, "Fire! Emergency! Somebody call 911!"

3. Monitor *Airway, Breathing,* and *Circulation.* Start CPR if the child is not breathing. (See page *24* for infants under one year of age; see page *41* for children aged one to eight.)

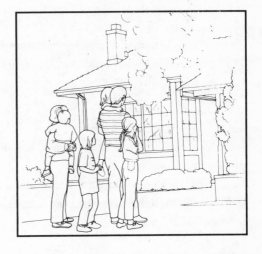

4. If a child has been confined to an enclosed, smoke-filled area call a physician if you do not have to call 911.

SUDDEN INFANT DEATH SYNDROME (SIDS)

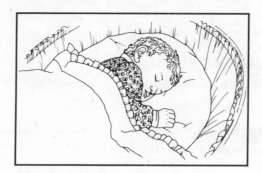

Sudden infant death syndrome (SIDS) is the sudden and unexplained death of a previously healthy baby for which no cause can be determined by autopsy. SIDS is also known as cot or crib death.

SIDS occurs in 1 out of every 500 to 600 live births and is the leading cause of death during the first year. The highest incidence of SIDS occurs during the winter months, in babies between two and six months of age. Although no one can predict which individuals will be affected, the incidence has been noted to be higher in certain groups, including:

- Babies born to mothers in methadone maintenance programs and to those using cocaine, especially when both drugs are taken
- Premature babies with chronic lung disease
- Babies with a low birth weight
- Siblings of babies who died of SIDS
- Babies of teenage mothers.

There is no way to prevent SIDS, because it cannot be predicted in individual babies and its exact cause is unknown.

If your baby has been identified as having risk factors for SIDS, you and your physician may decide to use a breathing monitor on your baby. The use of monitors is controversial, but they are still recommended for specific situations, determined on an individual basis.

If your baby nearly succumbs to SIDS—that is, he stops breathing, but is successfully resuscitated, or he experiences periods of apnea with or without blue skin color changes—notify your physician after intervening.

SYMPTOMS

- Unconsciousness without spontaneous breathing or pulse
- Blue color, especially in the mouth

TREATMENT

1. Start CPR. (See page *24* for infants under one year of age.) This may be a "near-miss SIDS event," or the breathing and heart may have stopped because of another problem.

2. Notify the fire and utilities departments nearest to your home if you have a child with special problems requiring an apnea monitor or oxygen.

3. If CPR is unsuccessful, support is essential. Many parents or caregivers feel that they were responsible for the SIDS event. Remember that babies have many capabilities to protect themselves, and SIDS is *not* caused by such things as having blankets or pillows in the crib. A healthy baby will turn his head or move a blanket from his face to breathe.

4. SIDS support groups are very helpful and are available in many places. Call your local hospital to find one close to you, or contact:

> The National SIDS Foundation
> 2 Metro Plaza, Suite 205
> 8240 Professional Place
> Landover, Maryland 20785

STRESS AND HOW TO REMEMBER WHAT YOU HAVE LEARNED

We realize that you may feel anxious after reading about all the potential emergencies that could affect your child. We do not wish to cause you to worry unnecessarily. You should feel good that you have taken the initiative to read this book, and you should feel some security in knowing how to manage an emergency problem.

Now is the time for you to take a CPR class in which you can practice your skills on a mannequin under the supervision of a certified instructor. When you call to ask about the classes, you should make certain that the instructors are certified to teach by the American Heart Association or by the American Red Cross.

You should also examine your home, school, or day-care center for potential hazards and remove them. Install necessary safety equipment such as smoke detectors and gates near stairs. Review *Safe & Sound* carefully to help you remember what changes you must make in the environment of your children.

We realize that we have given you much information and that the sequence of CPR and relief-of-choking skills can be difficult to remember. We encourage you to review the skills in your mind when you have time and, if you cannot remember what to do next, review *Safe & Sound*.

It is also a good idea to use mental imagery to prepare for an emergency. You might be in a store or on the street when something happens that might cause you to think about what you might have to do if an emergency arises. A child might be coughing in the store. You might imagine that the child stops coughing, cannot make a sound, and begins to turn blue. What would you do? Can you remember? Think about the order of the actions that you would take. Is there something that you could do to change your own environment to prevent the problem? If you forget something, find the answer in *Safe & Sound*.

If you prepare this way, your emergency care actions will become reflexive and you will act appropriately to care for your child. You can use the next few exercises to drill yourself or someone else.

Exercise 1:

You are in the park, when you suddenly hear a woman screaming that her child has fallen from the slide, hit his head, and is not moving. When you examine the child, you see that he is blue and not moving. What do you do? (Answer on pages *24–29 or 41–47.*)

Exercise 2:

You are at a party, and the children are playing upstairs. Someone goes to check on them because they are quiet, and calls out that two of the children took some pills. One is able to speak, but the other has collapsed and is not moving. What do you do? (Answer on pages *114–119.*)

Exercise 3:

You are walking down the street, and you see a child hit by a car. The child gets up and walks for a short distance, then falls. You approach the child and find that he is bleeding profusely from his leg. The blood is spurting. You start to help him and find that he is blue and has stopped breathing. What do you do? (Answer on pages *66–71.*)

Exercise 4:

You are in a toy store, and you hear an announcement that a child is choking in aisle thirteen. The employee is asking for help from anyone who knows CPR. You run to aisle thirteen and find a nine-month-old baby who is moving his arms, very agitated, and is unable to make any sound. He is trying to cry but no sound can be heard. What do you do? (Answer on pages *30–32.*)

Exercise 5:

You are at a crowded swimming pool. Suddenly someone shouts that his baby is drowning. Someone removes the two-year-old from the pool, and you see that he is blue and not moving. What do you do? (Answer on pages *79–83.*)

THE *SAFE & SOUND* BASIC FIRST-AID KIT

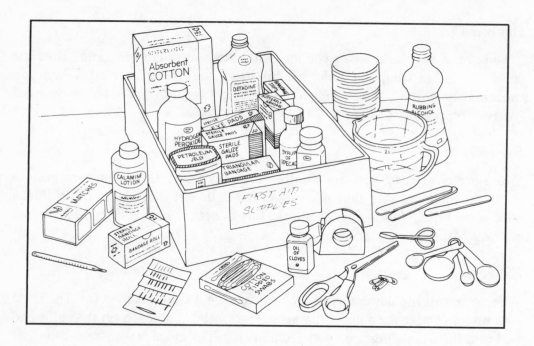

It is important to have at home a first-aid kit stocked with the items suggested below. Keep all supplies in a single box or container and store it in one place, out of reach of children but easily accessible to those caring for the children. A smaller kit can be kept in each car, and a separate kit should be taken on hiking or camping trips. Special snakebite kits and insect-sting kits are available to supplement your outdoor first-aid kit. Another kit should be kept aboard a boat. A kit complete with larger amounts of all items should be kept in every school and day-care center.

Commercial first-aid kits are available, but make sure to supplement them if they do not include all of the following items. Replace all supplies when used, old, or expired. Label each item and include its purpose if it is not obvious.

LIST OF SUPPLIES FOR A *SAFE & SOUND* FIRST-AID KIT

— Absorbent cotton
— Adhesive strip bandages of assorted sizes
— Adhesive tape, one-half to one inch wide (one to three centimeters)
— Betadine solution, for cleansing wounds
— Butterfly bandages
— Calamine lotion
— Children's aspirin substitute, as directed by your physician
— Cotton-tipped swabs
— Drinking cups (paper or plastic)
— Hydrogen peroxide, for cleansing wounds
— Large triangular bandages
— Matches
— Measuring cup
— Measuring spoons
— Oil of cloves, for minor toothache
— Petroleum jelly
— Phone numbers of doctor, ambulance, hospital, poison control center
— Rubbing alcohol
— Safety pins
— Sharp needles (sterilize first with a match before using to remove splinters)
— Sharp scissors
— Sterile bandage rolls of assorted sizes, one-half to two inches wide (one to five centimeters)
— Sterile eye pads
— Sterile gauze pads, two by two, two by four, and four by four inches (five by five, five by ten, and ten by ten centimeters)
— Syrup of ipecac (we recommend two bottles per child if your children are older than one year)
— Thermometer

THE *SAFE & SOUND* BASIC FIRST-AID KIT

___ Tongue depressors
___ Tourniquet (a clean cloth about two inches wide and twenty inches long—five centimeters wide, fifty centimeters long— or clean panty hose)
___ Tweezers

OTHER ITEMS THAT CAN BE USED DURING AN EMERGENCY

- Diapers, regular or disposable, can be used to control heavy bleeding and as bandages.
- Diaper pins can be used to pin bandages or slings.
- Large scarves can be used as eye bandages or slings.
- Magazines, newspapers, or umbrellas can be used as splints for broken bones.
- Panty hose, belts, or scarves can be used as tourniquets to control bleeding.
- A table leaf, coffee-table top, bookshelf, piano bench, ironing board, or old door can be used as a stretcher for head, neck, or back injuries.
- Towels, sheets, or tablecloths can be used to control bleeding and as bandages.

The purpose of *Safe & Sound* is to help you to learn how to manage life-threatening emergencies. We encourage you to read a general first-aid book to help you to manage minor problems. Special first-aid books for hiking and camping are also available. Always consult with your physician if you have any questions about minor problems. REMEMBER, IN AN EMERGENCY, CALL 911.

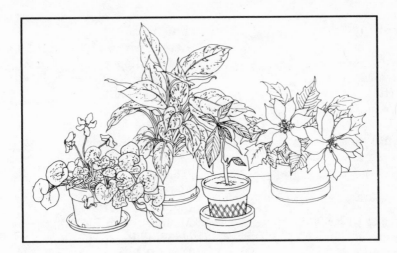

The following lists of nonpoisonous and poisonous plants are included to help you determine which plants in your environment are clearly dangerous. If your child likes to eat plants, or if you are not sure what type of plant you have, the best advice from experts is to remove the plant. *When in doubt, get it out!* Remember to call experts at the poison control center if you have questions, as well as during an emergency situation involving poisonous substances.

Nonpoisonous Plants

Abelia
Absynnian Sword Lily
African Daisy
African Palm
African Violet*
Airplane Plant
Air Plant
Aluminum Plant*
Aralia*
Araucaria
Aster
Baby's Breath or Baby's Tears*
Bachelor's Button

Bamboo
Begonia*
Bird's Nest Fern*
Bloodleaf Plant*
Boston Fern*
Bougainvillea
Bromeliad Family
Cactus (certain varieties)*
California Holly
California Poppy
Camellia
Chinese Evergreen*
Christmas Cactus

Coffee Tree
Coleus*
Corn Plant*
Crab Apples
Crape Myrtle
Creeping Jennie (Moneywort, Lysima)
Crocus
Croton (house variety)*
Dahlia
Dandelion
Dogwood
Donkey Tail*
Dragon Tree or Dracaena*
Easter Cactus
Easter Lily
Echeveria
Emerald Ripple
Eugenia
Fiddle-Leaf Fig
Fig Tree
Forget-Me-Not
Forsythia
Fuchsia
Gardenia
Geranium
Gloxinia
Grape Ivy*
Hawaiian Ti Plant
Hawthorn Berry
Heavenly Bamboo
Hedge Apples
Hibiscus
Honeysuckle
Hoya*
Ice Plant
Impatiens Walleriana
Jade Plant*
Jasmine

Kalanchoe
Lace Plant
Lady's Slipper
Lily (Day, Easter, or Tiger)*
Lily of the Nile
Lipstick Plant*
Magnolia
Maidenhair Fern*
Marigold
Monkey Plant
Moon Cactus
Mother of Pearls
Mountain Ash Berry
Nandina Berry
Natal Palm
Norfolk Island Pine
Old Man Cactus
Olive Tree
Orchid
Oregon Grape
Palm (Bamboo, Paradise, Parlor, Sentry)*
Pansy Flower
Passion Vine
Peanut Cactus
Pellionia
Peony Flower
Peperomia*
Petunia
Phlox
Piggy-back Plant*
Pigmy Date Palm
Pocketbook
Polka Dot Plant
Prayer Plant*
Purple Passion (Velvet Plant)*
Pussy Willow
Pyracantha Berry
Queen's Tears

Rabbit's Foot Fern
Rainbow Plant
Raphiolepsis
Rattlesnake Plant
Ribbon Plant
Rock Rose
Rosary Vine
Rosay Pearls
Roses
Rubber Plant*
Schefflera (Umbrella Plant)*
Sedum
Sensitive Plant*
Silver Heart
Snake Plant
Snapdragon
Spider Plant*
Staghorn Fern

Starfish Flower
String of Hearts
Swedish Ivy*
Sword Fern
Tahitian Bridal Veil
Umbrella Tree
Vagabond Plant
Velvet Plant
Venus's Flytrap
Violet
Wandering Jew*
Wax Plant
Weeping Fig*
Weeping Willow
Wild Onion
Yucca
Zebra Plant*
Zinnia

*Common houseplant

Poisonous Plants

Plants can be toxic in several ways. Some plant juices contain oxalates, which are irritating to the skin, mouth, and tongue, and which, in some cases, may cause stomach upset and breathing difficulties.

Some plants, if eaten, may cause nausea, vomiting, diarrhea, and/or abdominal cramps. Call your poison control center if any of these symptoms occurs. Other plants may cause a skin rash if contact occurs. If skin contacts occurs, wash the affected area with hand soap and water.

Acorn
Aloe vera*
Amaryllis
American Ivy
American Plum

Anemone
Angel's Trumpet
Anthurium
Apple (seeds)
Arrowhead Vine*

Asparagus Fern* (berry)
Avocado (leaves)
Azalea
Baneberry
Barberry
Betel Nut Palm
Bird of Paradise
Bittersweet
Black Locust
Bleeding Heart
Bloodroot
Blue Cohosh
Boston Ivy
Box, Boxwood
Buckeye
Bunchberry
Buttercup
Cactus (thorn)
Caladium
Calla Lily
Cardinal Flower
Carnation
Castor Bean
Century Plant
Choke Cherry
Christmas Rose
Chrysanthemum
Coral Berry
Cotoneaster
Creeping Charlie*
Crocus-Autumn, Meadow
Crown of Thorns
Cyclamen
Daffodil (bulb)
Daisy
Daphne
Deadly Nightshade
Death Camus

Delphinium
Devil's Ivy (Pothos)*
Dieffenbachia*
Dumb Cane
Elderberry
Elephant's Ear*
Emerald Duke
English Ivy*
Ficus Benjamina* (sap)
Four O'Clock
Foxglove
Garden Sorrel
Geranium, California
Glacier Ivy
Golden Chain
Ground Ivy
Heart Ivy
Heart Leaf
Henbane, Black
Hen and Chickens
Holly Berry
Horse Chestnut
Horse Nettle
Horsetail Reed
Hyacinth
Hydrangea
Inkberry
Iris
Ivy, American (berry)
Jack-in-the-Pulpit
Japanese Yew
Jequirity Bean
Jerusalem Cherry
Jessamine (note: *Jasmine* is
   nonpoisonous)
Jimson Weed (Thorn Apple)
Jonquil (bulb)
Juniper

Lantana Camera (Red Sage)
Larkspur
Laurel, English
Ligustrum Ovalifolium, Vulgare
Lily of the Valley
Lobelia
Locoweed
Majesty
Mandrake
Marble Queen
Marijuana
May Apple
Mistletoe, American*
Mistletoe, European
Monkshood
Moonseed
Morning Glory (seed)
Mushrooms (many wild varieties)
Narcissus
Nephthytis
Ohio Buckeye
Oleander
Parlor Ivy
Periwinkle
Peyote (Mescal)
Philodendron
Poinsettia*
Poison Hemlock (Fool's Parsley)
Poison Ivy
Poison Oak
Pokeweed
Poppy (except California)
Potato (green parts, sprouts)
Pothos
Primrose
Privet, Common/California

Prunus species (seed pits)
Pyracantha (berry and thorn)
Ranunculus
Red Sage
Rhododendron
Rhubarb (leaves)
Ripple Ivy
Rosary Bean/Pea
Saddleleaf
Seed Pits: Almond, Apple, Apricot
    Cherry, Peach, Pear, Plum
Shamrock Plant
Skunk Cabbage
Spathiphyllum
Split Leaf Philodendron
Sprengeri Fern
Squill
Star of Bethlehem
String of Beads/Pearls
Sweet Pea
Swiss Cheese Plant
Tobacco
Tomato (leaves)
Toyon (leaves)
Tulip (bulb)
Umbrella Plant
Vince
Virginia Creeper
Walnut (green shells)
Water Hemlock
White Locust
Wisteria
Wood-rose
Yew

*Common houseplant

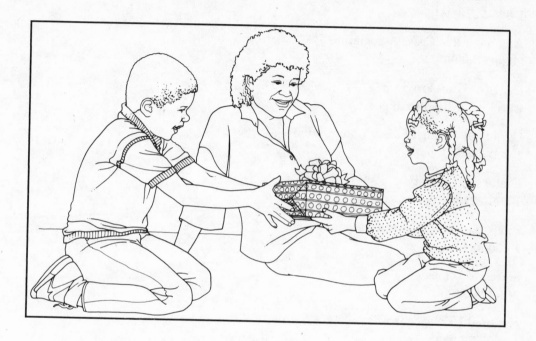

Children who feel stress can have accidents and illness more often than those who do not. It is important that children are supported and encouraged to grow and be creative, without being anxious or fatigued by feeling the need to be perfect. Your love and patient understanding of your children can provide them with the basis for a long, happy, and healthy life.

We hope that you now feel more secure by knowing the basic preventive measures and treatments for the most common childhood emergencies. One of the most important and responsible jobs in a society is caring for children. We recognize how tiring and demanding a job it is and hope that this book can assist those worthy people who protect the small and young ones.

American Automobile Association
1-800-652-1158

American Heart Association
1-800-527-6941

American Red Cross Association
202-639-6300

Car Seat Loan Program
Check your local listings

Consumer Product Safety Commission
1-800-638-7272

Easter Seal Society
1-800-221-6827

Environmental Protection Agency
1-800-424-9065

March of Dimes
914-428-7100

National Highway Traffic Safety Administration
1-800-424-9393

National Poison Center Network
412-647-5600

National SIDS Foundation
1-800-221-7437

National Trauma Society
1-800-759-7328

Pesticide Line
1-800-858-7378

Poison Control Center
1-800-662-9886

Sierra Club (for camping information)
202-547-1141

General Emergency: **911**

You are here: Name _____

Address _____

Near Major Street/Landmarks _____

Telephone _____

Poison Control Center: _____

Ambulance Company: _____

Fire Department: _____

Police: _____

Hospital Emergency Room: _____

Taxi: _____

Pediatrician: Name _____ Office _____ Home _____

Family Doctor: Name _____ Office _____ Home _____

Dentist: Name _____ Office _____ Home _____

Nearest Drugstore: _____ Hours _____ Telephone ____

24-hour Drugstore: _____ Telephone ____

Father's Telephone at Work: _____

Mother's Telephone at Work: _____

OTHER FAMILY MEMBERS

Name _____ Telephone _____

Name _____ Telephone _____

Name _____ Telephone _____

NEIGHBORS AND FRIENDS

Name _____ Telephone _____

Name _____ Telephone _____

Name _____ Telephone _____

Additional copies of *Safe & Sound* may be purchased from most booksellers or by mail on the order form below. Substantial discounts on orders of 10 or more copies are available to physicians, clinics, health-care providers, day-care centers, schools, and individuals. For information call:

St. Martin's Press
Special Sales Department
Toll Free (800) 221-7945
In New York State (212) 674-5151

	Copies	Price
Please send me _____ copies of *Safe & Sound* at $8.95 per copy ISBN: 0-312-02276-X	____	____
Postage and handling: $1.50 for first book and 75¢ for each additional book		____
Amount enclosed		____

Name: _____

Address: _____

City/State/Zip: _____

Send this form with payment to St. Martin's Press / Cash Sales Dept. / 175 Fifth Avenue / New York, NY 10010. Please allow three weeks for delivery.